——— THE ULTIMATE GUIDE TO ———

SUGARS & SWEETENERS

Dear Peter,

I hope you enjoy!

[signature]

THE EXPERIMENT

BECAUSE EVERY BOOK IS A TEST OF NEW IDEAS

THE ULTIMATE GUIDE TO

SUGARS & SWEETENERS

Discover the Taste, Use, Nutrition, Science, and Lore of Everything from Agave Nectar to Xylitol

ALAN BARCLAY, PHD, PHILIPPA SANDALL, AND CLAUDIA SHWIDE-SLAVIN, MS, RD, CDE

THE EXPERIMENT

NEW YORK

The Experiment, LLC
220 East 23rd Street, Suite 301
New York, NY 10010-4674
www.theexperimentpublishing.com

This book contains the opinions and ideas of its authors. It is intended to provide helpful and informative material on the subjects addressed in the book. It is sold with the understanding that the authors and publisher are not engaged in rendering medical, health, or any other kind of personal professional services in the book. The authors and publisher specifically disclaim all responsibility for any liability, loss, or risk—personal or otherwise—that is incurred as a consequence, directly or indirectly, of the use and application of any of the contents of this book.

The Experiment's books are available at special discounts when purchased in bulk for premiums and sales promotions as well as for fund-raising or educational use. For details, contact us at info@theexperimentpublishing.com.

Library of Congress Cataloging-in-Publication Data
Barclay, Alan W.
  The ultimate guide to sugars and sweeteners : discover the taste, use, nutrition, science, and lore of everything from agave nectar to xylitol / Alan Barclay, PhD, Philippa Sandall, and Claudia Shwide-Slavin, MS, RD, CDE.
    pages cm
  Includes bibliographical references and index.
  ISBN 978-1-61519-216-8 (pbk.) -- ISBN 978-1-61519-217-5 (ebook) 1. Sweeteners. I. Sandall, Philippa. II. Shwide-Slavin, Claudia. III. Title.
  TP421.B37 2014
  664'.1--dc23
                    2014027435

ISBN 978-1-61519-216-8
Ebook ISBN 978-1-61519-217-5

Cover design by Christopher Brian King
Cover photographs © StockFood/Richard Jung Photography
Text design by Pauline Neuwirth, Neuwirth & Associates, Inc.

Manufactured in the United States of America
Distributed by Workman Publishing Company, Inc.
Distributed simultaneously in Canada by Thomas Allen & Son Ltd.
First printing November 2014
10 9 8 7 6 5 4 3 2 1

CONTENTS

FOREWORD

My guess is that many of you reading this book are trying to improve your dietary habits. No doubt, high on your to-do list is cutting down on "sugar" (the stuff described as pure, white, and deadly). But I will hazard another guess: you haven't cut all sweetness out of your life—you've just exchanged one source of sweetness for another. Now you're wondering, is the new source a good one, a better one, or actually doing more harm than good? Well, that's exactly why Alan Barclay, Philippa Sandall, and Claudia Shwide-Slavin wrote *The Ultimate Guide to Sugars and Sweeteners*. To my knowledge, they are the first to bring all this information altogether in one consumer-friendly, very readable little book. They've done the hard work for you. They tell you not only what each sugar or sweetener is and where it comes from, but also its history, chemistry, calorie content, culinary applications, and—wherever they can—its effect on blood glucose (in other words, its glycemic index).

I expect many of you will find it surprising to hear a professor of nutrition express the view that sugars and sweeteners have a place in modern diets. Perhaps it comes from a university training in food science, combined with a passionate interest in diet and human evolution. A diet with a moderate amount of added sugars (about 5 to 10 percent of total energy, or 25 to 50 grams in a 2,000-calorie diet) is the amount considered commensurate with a nutritious diet by the World Health Organization. I don't believe that it's helpful to strictly avoid all sources of added sugars.

Why? For one, it's highly likely that you'll replace those calories with something else. Not at a conscious level, of course, but in the appetite center of your brain, hormones and other signals will ensure you're maintaining your usual body weight.

Research shows us that if you cut sugar calories from your diet, there's a good chance you'll eat more calories from fat, particularly saturated fat (the so-called sugar-fat seesaw). Consuming more saturated fat will definitely increase your risk of chronic disease. If you're careful to avoid both saturated fat and added sugars, perhaps you'll eat more refined fats and oils that are also "empty calories," just like added sugars. So you'll have achieved nothing.

Or perhaps you'll eat more starch, particularly the highly refined starches that are also empty calories and contribute to a high dietary glycemic load (think your typical French fries, white rice, white bread, and highly processed breakfast cereals). These foods raise blood glucose more than other sources of carbohydrates, and they also increase the risk of chronic disease. And there's a good chance you'll consume more salt, too, because starchy foods are bland without it.

Concentrated sources of sugars have a long history as part of our diet. Sugars in fruit and honey have provided carbohydrate energy in human diets for millions of years—ever since primates began evolving on a steady diet of fruit and berries in the rainforests of Africa fifty million years ago. The appreciation of the sensation of sweetness runs deep in the human psyche. Our hunter-gatherer ancestors positively relished concentrated sugars such as dates, dried fruit, sugar bag, honey, and even honey ants. In literature and mythology, sweetness is linked with pleasure and goodness, and in everyday language we use terms associated with sweetness to describe the things we love (sweetie pie, honeymoon). Our first food, breast milk, is sweet—in fact, it's the sweetest of all mammalian milks.

We should, therefore, use added sugars judiciously to increase the intake of nutritious foods that might otherwise not appeal (think a little melted brown sugar on hot oatmeal, a swirl of date syrup on yogurt). With this thought in mind, I recommend this A-to-Z guide as the best, most up-to-date, and accurate source of information about all the sugars and sweeteners, new and old, in our diet.

Jennie Brand-Miller, PhD, author of the Low GI Diet Revolution series and Professor of Nutrition and Metabolism, School of Molecular Bioscience and Charles Perkins Centre, University of Sydney, Australia

April 2014

INTRODUCTION:
SEEKING SWEETNESS

Our sweet tooth has a long history. It seems we have always been drawn to sweet things, but supply was generally limited, unreliable, and seasonal—until now.

Today, many anthropologists believe that honey is one of the sweet secrets to human evolution and that for thousands of years our diet has included a variety of natural sugars from fruits, berries, saps, gums, leaf scale, honey ants, nectar, and honeycomb. Seeking sweetness made sense for early humans, whose energy-hungry, expanding brains would have greatly benefited from the calories and nourishment these sweet foods provided, especially when the hunter came home empty-handed. The earliest evidence we have for seeking sweetness is in rock art by our hunter-gatherer ancestors from all around the world that depicts honeycombs, swarms of bees, and honey collecting and that date back thousands of years. But there is also potentially older evidence in the mutually beneficial relationship between the honeyguide bird and the hunter-gatherer in Africa.

Today, most of us buy our honey in jars from shops, but some Hadza, who live near Lake Eyasi in northern Tanzania, don't. They haven't settled down to village or town life. They are mobile foragers who still hunt honey (their number one preferred food item) as their ancestors did for thousands of years. And, like their ancestors, they sometimes seek it with the assistance of the aptly named honeyguide bird (*Indicator indicator*):

The honeyguide bird and the human honey hunter communicate through a series of whistles, and the bird guides the hunter, tree by tree, to the hive. Once the honey hunter has located the hive, he pounds wooden pegs into the trunk of the tree, climbs to the top where the hive is located, chops into the tree to expose the hive, and smokes it out by placing burning brush into the opening. Smoking the hive acts to pacify the bees by dulling the senses of the guard bees, who protect the opening of the hive. The bees see the smoke as a habitat threat and focus on collecting enough honey to rebuild their hive elsewhere. This allows the hunter to collect the honeycomb without being stung by the killer bees. The honeyguide bird patiently waits outside of the hive, and as the honey hunter obtains his honeycomb prize, the honeyguide bird is rewarded with its delicious prize— wax from the comb and bees.[1]

In our own lives, our first taste of life is sweetness: mother's milk, the food that Mother Nature designed for our babies. It contains the sugar lactose, and it is the sweetest of all mammalian milks. (The nutrients in baby formulas are matched to it as closely as possible, but it is hard to match breast milk's natural sweetness without adding some kind of sweetener.) Research shows that new babies prefer sweet tastes from birth. They will choose to suck on bottles of sweetened water but will turn away or cry if given something bitter or sour to taste. The appealing sweetness of the lactose in breast milk is part of a perfect nutritional package containing all the proteins, fats, vitamins, and minerals that babies need to grow and thrive and fight infection.

The take-home lesson is that adding a sprinkle of sugar or a drizzle of honey can be a great way to encourage us to eat healthy foods. A touch of sweetness helps us enjoy nutritious foods such as oatmeal (porridge) and plain yogurt. The Academy of Nutrition and Dietetics advises that "Consumers can safely enjoy a range of nutritive sweeteners and nonnutritive [zero-calorie] sweeteners when consumed within an eating plan that is guided by current federal nutrition recommendations, such as the Dietary Guidelines for Americans and the Dietary Reference Intakes, as well as individual health goals and personal preference."[2]

But, naturally appealing or not, nutritive sugars and sweeteners such as honey are not health foods, because they provide us with energy (calories/kilojoules) but not much else in the way of nutritional benefits. So, we most certainly are not going to encourage you to consume as much as you'd like. Moderation matters if you want to achieve and maintain a healthy weight. What's moderate? Currently, the World Health Organization (WHO) recommends that people should not eat more than 10 percent of their total daily calories from added sugars. For a typical American adult consuming 2,000 calories a day, this is equal to around 12 teaspoons—200 calories. This is based on an observation in epidemiological studies that the risk of developing tooth decay increases when a population's average consumption of added sugar (that is, sugar not occurring naturally in foods) goes above 10 percent of their calorie intake. (We show you what 10 percent added sugars look like in Part 2, on page 215.) The WHO's new draft guidelines as of March 2014 also say that consuming less than 5 percent of total calories from added sugars may provide additional health benefits.[3]

When cutting back on added sugars, the food industry and many consumers turn to nonnutritive sweeteners. However, if you are trying to cut calories, it's important to remember that "sugar-free" isn't code for "low calorie." When regular sugar is replaced by ▶**nonnutritive sweeteners** in energy-dense (high-calorie) starchy or fatty foods, you may not save very many calories at all.

Controversy swirls around nonnutritive sweeteners' safety: you have likely heard rumors that one or more of these sweeteners is toxic, carcinogenic, or otherwise harmful. In the entries in this book, we will not address specific claims about various sweeteners' toxicity, because the rigorous clinical evidence that regulatory agencies such as the US Food and Drug Administration (FDA) take into account when approving sweeteners and other food additives does not support those claims—at least, not in the quantities we can reasonably expect someone to consume. If you have concerns about specific sweeteners' safety, we suggest you visit the website of the regulatory body for your country, which not only is responsible for the rigorous approval process but also continues to closely monitor and review new evidence about these additives on an ongoing basis. You will find, for example, that the FDA's latest review of studies focused on ▶**aspartame** found no evidence that it contributes to developing cancer. See the entry on nonnutritive sweeteners for more details and website links.

There's no question that these days, there is a lot of confusion about sugars and sweeteners. The science can be complicated, and researchers and various other self-appointed "experts" whose claims get media attention seem to contradict one another about what's okay and what's not. It is hard for the average consumer to sort fact from fiction. But there's also a great deal that we *do* know about sugars and sweeteners and what happens when we consume them, thanks to evidence-based scientific research that does not always make headlines. We wrote this book to share the evidence with you. And we have to confess, we have had great fun trying out a wide range of traditional sugars and syrups from around the world. We have discovered how delicious tahini with a drizzle of date syrup is, for example.

We also have a website, sugarsandsweeteners.com, where we post stories to keep you up-to-date on the latest research on sugars and sweeteners and on new products to hit the market.

Rest assured, we aren't out to change your mind or your dietary habits (unless you want to). We are out to give you the most accurate information on sugars and sweeteners (nutritive—the ones with calories—and nonnutritive—the ones without calories) to help you make the best possible choices for your health when it comes to shopping, cooking, and dining out; as well as for taste, texture, sweetness, and performance in recipes; and for environmental and ethical reasons if they concern you. We also want you to have this information so that you can share it, perhaps playing a part in correcting the tsunami of misinformation about sugars and sweeteners. Studies suggest that people who understand the science, history, and production process of an ingredient are smarter, savvier consumers.[4] We hope this book helps you to make smart, savvy choices in your moderately sweet daily life.

ABOUT USING THIS BOOK

To make the information as accessible as possible, the main alphabetical entries on sugars and sweeteners in Part 1 follow a similar structure:

NAME

(Alternative names)

Description, including appropriate ▶**cross references** and substitution tips.

▶ **AT A GLANCE** summary to give you the fast facts you need to know.
   For nutritive sweeteners (the ones that provide calories/kilojoules) they include:

Nutritive
Sugars tells you which sugars the sweetener contains—e.g., fructose, glucose, sucrose
Sweetness relative to sucrose
Calories (kilojoules) per level teaspoon
Health includes specific health concerns pertaining to a sweetener (e.g., warnings for those with certain health conditions or who are pregnant or breastfeeding); more general health information appears in Part 2, page 209

For nonnutritive sweeteners (the ones that don't provide calories/ kilojoules) they include:

Nonnutritive

Sweetness relative to sucrose

Calories

FDA approval

EFSA Number

ADI tells you the Acceptable Daily Intake per kilogram (2.2 pounds) of body weight per day; see page 9 for more details

LTV tells you the Laxative Threshold Value and appears only if the sweetener has laxative properties; see page 11 for more details

Health includes specific health concerns pertaining to a sweetener (e.g., warnings for those with certain health conditions or who are pregnant or breastfeeding); more general health information appears in Part 2, page 209

In Part 2 we look at sugars, sweeteners, and health, with topics including added sugars, dietary guidelines, digestion and absorption of sugars and sweeteners, tooth decay, diabetes, heart diseases, weight gain, special diets such as gluten-free or low-FODMAP, and regulations regarding the labeling of sugars and sweeteners.

Part 3 is for those who love baking. We commissioned Chrissy Freer to report on how some of the most popular sweeteners measured up compared with granulated white sugar in baking a Vanilla Butter Cookie and Blueberry Bran Muffin.

To entertain, inform and round out the story, we have included:

- BUZZ NOTES (or fact boxes) featuring snippets of science, ethnography, botany, biology, history, lore, and trivia
- Q&As to give you the answers to the most frequently asked questions about sugars and sweeteners

To help you find what you are looking for as quickly as possible, the first time in any entry where the name of another entry is used, you will find it marked this way: ▶**aspartame**. When we refer to information other than entries, we provide page numbers.

Before you begin, check out our glossary of acronyms (page 9) and the basic science behind the glycemic index (page 12).

MEASURING AND COUNTING

CALORIES AND KILOJOULES

One gram of carbohydrates (that's sugars and starches) contains 4 calories or 17 kilojoules (there are 4.2 kilojoules in 1 calorie). How does that compare with protein and fat? 1 gram of protein also contains 4 calories (17 kilojoules); 1 gram of alcohol contains 7 calories (29 kilojoules); 1 gram of fat contains 9 calories (37 kilojoules). Remember, calories and kilojoules are not a measure of a food's quality or whether or not it is good for you, but of its energy content.

NUTRITION ANALYSIS

We sourced our nutrient data from the USDA and FSANZ databases. In select cases, when products were not included in these databases, we used nutrient information from manufacturers.

MEASURING

The teaspoon we refer to in this book for counting calories and grams of carbohydrates (and for measuring in the recipes) is not the silver teaspoon in your cutlery drawer; it is the standard teaspoon you find in a set of measuring spoons, and it is level (not heaped). One level teaspoon is equivalent to 5 milliliters (ml) and contains 4.2 grams (g) of available (digestible) carbohydrates (which excludes fiber). As this is not the most user-friendly number for mental math, it is standard practice in nutrition tables to round it down to 4 grams, and that is what we have done throughout the book to be consistent. However, you will find that some manufacturers round up to 5 grams on nutrition labels (and we think this is a good idea, as most people don't use measuring spoons when adding sugar to their tea—and even if they do, they probably don't use level ones).

DAY-TO-DAY MEASURING AND COUNTING

Nutrient data is based on level measures (teaspoons, tablespoons, and cups). While many of us will level off a cup measure in cooking and baking for optimal results, few of us will bother to level off a teaspoon of sugar with the back of a knife. But for day-to-day measuring and counting, you should allow for the fact that the teaspoon of sugar you stir into a cup of tea or coffee is probably rounded or heaping (equivalent to about 1½ teaspoons) and therefore has more calories than you thought. Check out the difference (measures rounded):

MEASURE (GRANULATED SUGAR)	CALORIES	KILOJOULES	GRAMS
1 level teaspoon (5 ml)	16	67	4
1 rounded or heaping teaspoon = 1½ teaspoons (7.5 ml)	24	100	6
1 level tablespoon (15 ml)	48	201	12
1 rounded or heaping tablespoon= 1½ tablespoons (22.5 ml)	72	302	18
1 level Australian tablespoon (20 ml)	64	268	16
1 rounded or heaping Australian tablespoon= 1½ tablespoons (30 ml)	96	403	24

WHAT ACRONYM IS THAT?

ADI (ACCEPTABLE DAILY INTAKE)

The ADI is the amount of a specific food additive established as safe to consume per day. When regulatory food authorities evaluate sugar substitutes and sweeteners as additives for our food supply, they usually set an ADI. The figure is a conservative estimate based on the best available evidence of how much any person can safely consume each day over a lifetime. It includes a hundredfold safety margin, meaning that when the additive was tested in the lab, even an amount of the additive 100 times the ADI yielded no observable toxic effects.

In the United States, the Food and Drug Administration (FDA) sets the ADI; in other countries it is established by the Joint FAO (Food and Agriculture Organization of the UN)/WHO (World Health Organization) Expert Committee on Food Additives (JECFA) and the European Food Safety Authority (EFSA).

To work out how many cans of diet soda or packets of a nonnutritive sweetener you can safely consume each day, check the Acceptable Daily Intake Calculator of Noncaloric Sweeteners at nafwa.org/sweetener.php.

EFSA (EUROPEAN FOOD SAFETY AUTHORITY)

The European Food Safety Authority is an independent European agency funded by the EU budget that provides independent scientific advice and is the keystone of European Union risk assessment regarding food safety. See specific details about sweeteners at the EFSA website: efsa.europa.eu/en/topics/topic/sweeteners.htm.

E NUMBERS (EUROPEAN FOOD SAFETY AUTHORITY NUMBERS)

In the European Union all food additives are identified by an E number. Product labels must identify both the function of the additive in the finished food (e.g., "sweetener") and the specific substance used either by referring to the appropriate E number or its name (e.g., E950 or ▶**acesulfame potassium**). You will find E numbers on food labels on packaged foods sold within the European Union and Switzerland, the Cooperation Council for the Arab States of the Gulf, Australia, New Zealand, and Israel. They are occasionally found on North American packaging on imported European products.

The full list of E numbers covers:

- Colors (E100–E199)
- Preservatives (E200–E299)
- Antioxidants, acidity regulators (E300–E399)
- Thickeners, stabilizers, emulsifiers (E400–E499)
- Acidity regulators, anticaking agents (E500–E599)
- Flavor enhancers (E600–E699)
- Antibiotics (E700–E799)
- Glazing agents and sweeteners (E900–E999)
- Additional chemicals (E1000–E1599)

Where applicable, we have included EFSA numbers for sweeteners used as food additives.

FDA (FOOD AND DRUG ADMINISTRATION)

The Food and Drug Administration (United States) is an agency within the Department of Health and Human Services that is responsible for protecting and promoting public health through the regulation and supervision of food safety. It also regulates tobacco products, dietary supplements, prescription and over-the-counter pharmaceutical drugs (medications), vaccines, biopharmaceuticals, blood transfusions, medical devices, electromagnetic radiation emitting devices (ERED), cosmetics, and veterinary products.

See specific details about sweeteners at the FDA website: fda.gov/food/ingredientspackaginglabeling/foodadditivesingredients/ucm397725.htm.

FSANZ (FOOD STANDARDS AUSTRALIA AND NEW ZEALAND)

Food Standards Australia and New Zealand is a bi-national government agency that develops and administers the Australia New Zealand

Food Standards Code, which lists requirements for foods such as additives, food safety, labeling, and genetically modified foods. See specific details about sweeteners at the FSANZ website: foodstandards.gov.au/consumer/additives/intensesweetener/Pages/default.aspx.

GRAS (GENERALLY RECOGNIZED AS SAFE)

Before a sugar substitute or sweetener can be legally added to a food or beverage in United States, it must either have FDA approval or be accepted as GRAS (Generally Recognized As Safe).

GRAS dates back to 1959, when the FDA established a list of food substances that were exempt from the then-new requirement that manufacturers test food additives before putting them on the market. It includes "any substance that is intentionally added to food . . . generally recognized, among qualified experts, as having been adequately shown to be safe under the conditions of its intended use."[5]

Manufacturers can "self-affirm" the GRAS status of food additives they use in their products. Based on evidence of safety recognized by qualified experts, the manufacturer notifies the FDA that a particular use of a substance (in foods or beverages) is GRAS. If the FDA agrees, it issues a "No Objection" letter. It goes without saying that additives are continually being reevaluated based on the latest evidence. Sweeteners with GRAS status in the United States include ▶**stevia** (steviol glycosides) and most ▶**polyols** (sugar alcohols).

JECFA (JOINT FAO/WHO EXPERT COMMITTEE ON FOOD ADDITIVES)

This is an international scientific committee that evaluates food additive safety and is administered by the Food and Agriculture Organization (FAO) and the World Health Organization (WHO).

LTV (LAXATIVE THRESHOLD VALUE)

When sweeteners are evaluated as food additives, regulatory authorities also determine, where appropriate, the LTV. This is the amount that may cause a laxative effect if consumed over the course of a day or in a single meal. This is particularly relevant to ▶**polyols** (sugar alcohols).

UNDERSTANDING THE GLYCEMIC INDEX (GI) AND WHY IT MATTERS

W e have a number of handy tools in our healthy-eating tool kit to help us compare one food with another and make better choices when shopping, preparing family meals, and eating out. For example, the calorie (kilojoule) is a measure we routinely apply to food (which you now find on menus in many fast food restaurants). It measures the amount of energy in a portion of food. Although most people would probably struggle to explain exactly what a calorie (kilocalorie, to be precise) is, they know that calories count and that the quantity of calories they consume is a key factor in what they wind up weighing, especially if they aren't very active. The higher the number of calories we regularly consume each day, the higher the number on the bathroom scale is likely to be.

GLYCEMIC INDEX (GI)

The glycemic index (usually abbreviated to GI), is another handy measure. It is simply a number (typically between 1 and 100) that gives us a good indication of how fast our body is going to digest, absorb, and metabolize foods containing carbohydrates. Think of it as a speedometer that measures how fast and high your ▶**blood glucose** level (BGL) is likely to rise after you consume ▶**carbohydrate**-rich foods and beverages such as breads, cereals, grains, rice, noodles, pasta, fruit, starchy vegetables (e.g., potatoes, corn, sweet potatoes, or peas), legumes (e.g., lentils, chickpeas, and other beans), milk, yogurt, fries, chips, other similar savory snacks, cakes, cookies, sugars, and sweeteners.

When we consume these sorts of foods, our bodies convert the sugars and ▶**starches** (carbohydrates) in them to ▶**glucose** to fuel our brains, cells, tissues, and muscles (particularly during strenuous exercise), but it converts them at very different rates. Some foods break down quickly during digestion ("gushers"), and the glucose in

our blood increases rapidly; others break down slowly during digestion, and the glucose is released gradually into the blood ("tricklers").
And, of course, there are moderates in between.

The glycemic index is simply the measure that tells us which food
will do what. It has to be measured in people (we call it *in vivo* testing),
not in test tubes (*in vitro* testing), according to an internationally standardized method. High-glycemic-index foods and beverages have a GI
of 70 and above; moderate-glycemic-index foods and beverages have a
GI between 56 and 69; and low-glycemic-index foods and beverages
have a GI of 55 and under. With sugary foods that contain glucose,
▶**fructose**, ▶**lactose**, ▶**maltose**, or ▶**sucrose**, we can make educated
guesses as to whether they are likely to be high, moderate, or low glycemic index. It's much harder to estimate with starchy foods. Here's why:

Sugars and foods containing sugars

The glycemic index of sugars ranges from GI 19 for fructose to GI 46
for lactose, GI 65 for sucrose, GI 100 for glucose, and GI 105 for
maltose—a fivefold difference between fructose and maltose. Most
fruit-based products (fresh, dried, and canned fruit and fruit juices)
and dairy foods have a low glycemic index, because the predominant
carbohydrates (the sugars fructose and ▶**galactose**) in these products have a low glycemic index. On the other hand, most foods and
beverages made primarily from ▶**granulated sugar** (sucrose), such
as sweets and soft drinks, have a medium glycemic index—not high,
as is often assumed. Of course, unlike fruit and dairy foods, soft
drinks and sweets are occasional treats (not everyday foods); even if
the balance of sugars was changed to lower their glycemic index,
they would still contain no nutrients other than carbohydrates.

Starchy foods

For a variety of reasons, the type of starch contained in a food is
not as strong a predictor of its glycemic index as is the type of
sugar. There are two main types of starch—amylopectin and
amylose, which has the lower glycemic index. However, although a
food higher in amylose might have a lower glycemic index than
one higher in amylopectin, this is not always the case. This is
partly because the starches in unrefined grains, such as hulled barley, brown rice, or wheat berries, are encapsulated by the germ and
bran, which, when left intact, can make the starch—regardless of

type—very hard to digest. Of course, this is why we process them to provide us with more digestible forms (e.g., pearl barley, white rice, and bulgur, or flour).

Research has shown that the milling method (e.g., stone grinding versus modern steel roller milling) generally has a significant effect on the ultimate glycemic index of grain foods. Traditional stone-ground flours retain much more of the germ and bran and have more coarsely ground endosperm (where the starch is found), so the starch is still much harder to digest than that of modern roller-milled grains, giving it a lower glycemic index value.

Okay, you say, got all that, but why does it matter how high our blood glucose level is raised?
As with our blood pressure, there's a healthy range and a risky range. Having blood glucose levels over the day in the normal range is good for our bodies because it also lowers our daylong insulin levels. Here's what happens: As our BGL rises after a meal or a snack, our pancreas gets the message to release insulin, the powerful hormone that helps move the glucose out of the blood and into the cells. Having high blood glucose levels over the day from eating too many high-glycemic-index foods can put pressure on your health, because it means that the pancreas has to work extra hard producing more insulin to move the glucose into the cells, where it provides energy for the body and brain. Research around the world now shows that switching to eating mainly low-GI carbs that slowly trickle glucose into your bloodstream lowers your daylong blood glucose and insulin levels. These beneficial changes will:

- Help you control your appetite because you will feel fuller for longer
- Maximize your muscle mass
- Minimize your body fat
- Decrease your risk of heart disease and type 2 diabetes.

Remember, like calories, the glycemic index is a dietary tool. It's our responsibility to use both these tools to make healthier food choices, keep our portions moderate, and push back from the table when we have eaten enough.

GLYCEMIC LOAD (GL)

How high your ▶**blood glucose** actually rises and how long it remains high after you eat a meal containing ▶**carbohydrates** depends on both the amount of carbohydrates in the meal and the carbohydrates' glycemic index. Researchers from Harvard University and the University of Toronto came up with a term to describe this combination: glycemic load (GL). It is calculated by multiplying the GI of a food by the available carbohydrate content (carbohydrates minus ▶**fiber**) in the serving (expressed in grams), divided by 100 (because GI is a percent). (GL = GI/100 x available carbs per serving.)

For example, a typical medium-size apple has a glycemic index of 38 and contains 15 grams of available carbohydrate. Therefore, its glycemic load is 38 × 15 ÷ 100 = 6. If you are hungry, and the apples are particularly crispy, juicy, and delicious, so you eat two, the overall glycemic load of this snack is 12.

One unit of glycemic load is equivalent to 1 gram of pure ▶**glucose**. So, the higher the glycemic load of a food or meal, the more insulin your pancreas needs to produce to drive the glucose into your cells. When you are young, your pancreas is able to produce enough insulin to cover the requirements of high-glycemic-load foods and meals, but as you get older, it may no longer be able to cope with higher insulin requirements. This is when type 2 diabetes and other "lifestyle" diseases can start to develop.

In the GI and GL Table of Nutritive Sugars and Sweeteners on page 16, we show you the difference in the GL between 1 level teaspoon and 1 level tablespoon of these foods.

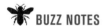 **BUZZ NOTES**

Glycemic Index (GI) and Glycemic Load (GL) of Nutritive Sugars and Sweeteners

We sourced the glycemic index values for this table from the International Tables of GI and GL Values and the free online database at glycemicindex .com maintained by the Sydney University Glycemic Index Research Service.[6] The sugars, sweeteners, and syrups listed here have been tested using the internationally standardized method.

In 1 level teaspoon, there are actually 4.2 grams of available ▶**carbohydrates** (net carbs) as we mentioned in the Introduction. As this is not the most user-friendly number for mental math, it is standard practice in nutrition to round the amount down to 4. We have also followed standard practice in rounding up and down the glycemic load values.

GI AND GL TABLE OF NUTRITIVE SUGARS AND SWEETENERS

SUGAR OR SWEETENER	GI	AVAILABLE CARBS– PER LEVEL TEASPOON (GRAMS)	GL 1 LEVEL TEASPOON	GL 1 LEVEL (15 ML) TABLESPOON	GL 1 LEVEL (20 ML) TABLESPOON (AUSTRALIA/ NEW ZEALAND)
Agave nectar or syrup	19–28	4	1	2–3	3–4
Coconut sugar	54	4	2	6	8
Corn syrup (dark)	90	4	4	12	16
Fructose	19	4	1	2	3
Glucose	100	4	4	12	16
Golden syrup	63	4	3	9	12
Grape syrup	52	4	2	6	8
Honey	32–87	4	2–3.5	6–11	8–14
Isomalt	2	5	0	0	0
Lactose	46	5	2	6	8
Maltose	105	5	5	16	21
Maltitol	26	5	1	4	5
Maple syrup	54	4	2	6	8
Molasses (treacle)	68	4	3	9	12
Polydextrose (Litesse: polydextrose with sorbitol)	7	5	0	1	1
Rice syrup	98	4	4	12	16
Sugar, granulated	65 (avg.)	4	3	9	12
Xylitol	21	5	1	3	4

What about nonnutritive sweeteners?

High-intensity, nonnutritive sweeteners such as ▶**acesulfame potassium**, ▶**alitame**, ▶**aspartame**, ▶**cyclamate**, ▶**monk fruit (luo han guo)**, ▶**neotame**, ▶**saccharin**, ▶**stevia**, ▶**sucralose**, and ▶**thaumatin** have virtually no effect on ▶**blood glucose** levels because most are used in such small quantities (providing insignificant, if any, calories and other nutrients) and are generally either not absorbed or not metabolized by the body. Some sources, therefore, list the GI as 0, but this has not been tested.

PART

1

SUGARS & SWEETENERS

A TO Z

ACESULFAME POTASSIUM

(aceK, acesulfame K; see brand names on page 270)

Science is filled with moments of serendipity, when researchers looking for one thing discover something completely different that ends up being far more profitable in the long run, although not necessarily for them. These moments have been very much a part of the ▶**nonnutritive (zero-calorie) sweetener** story. The discoveries of ▶**saccharin** (1879), ▶**cyclamate** (1937), ▶**aspartame** (1965), acesulfame potassium (1967), and ▶**sucralose** (1976) were all such "happy accidents."

Karl Clauss discovered acesulfame potassium when he was working at Hoechst (now Nutrinova, a global manufacturer of food components) and licked his fingers to pick up a piece of paper lying on the laboratory counter, inadvertently getting his first, surprisingly sweet taste of acesulfame potassium. The rest, as they say, is history. He gets the claim to fame and Nutrinova the patents for this zero-calorie, zero-carbohydrate, ▶**high-intensity sweetener** that is around 200 times sweeter than regular white ▶**granulated sugar (▶sucrose)**.

The name may not be quite as familiar as aspartame, but acesulfame potassium can be found in most aisles of the supermarket in thousands of food, beverage, oral-hygiene, and pharmaceutical products. Because one sweetener can mask another's aftertaste, acesulfame potassium is typically blended with other sweeteners (often aspartame) to provide the right type of sweetness for the product. In addition to tabletop products for sweetening tea or coffee, it is widely used in diet and so-called "diabetic-friendly" products (gum, soft drinks, yogurts, puddings, baked goods, canned foods, candies) and in mouthwashes. Like the proverbial "spoonful of sugar," it also helps the medicine go down by making chewable and liquid medications more palatable.

Chemically, this white crystalline powder is a potassium salt. "K" is the symbol for the chemical element potassium. Because "acesulfame potassium" is a bit of a mouthful, it is often abbreviated to aceK, which sounds more consumer friendly. Acesulfame potassium is what is called a nonnutritive sweetener, which simply means that it doesn't provide any calories (energy) because it has no nutrients (e.g., protein, carbohydrates, or fat) and no effect on ▶**blood glucose** levels. Nor does it influence potassium intake, despite being a potassium salt, because it passes through the body, is excreted in urine, and gets flushed away without being metabolized.

Being heat stable, acesulfame potassium is suitable for using in cooking and baking, though you may want to try it in one of the manufacturer's recipes before substituting it for sugar in your own favorites. The website for one brand of acesulfame potassium, Sweet One® (sweetone.com) explains that a 1-gram packet of Sweet One® contains the equivalent sweetness of two teaspoons of sugar, but the sweetness does not increase proportionately in cooking and baking. Alongside specific recipes and a substitution chart, the site provides these general tips:

- In sweetened sauces and beverages, replace all the granulated sugar with it.
- In baked goods, replace half of the specified amount of granulated sugar with it, because sugar provides baking with bulk, structure, moisture, and color as well as sweetness. For example, the Oatmeal Raisin Cookies recipe on the Sweet One® website calls for ⅓ cup granulated sugar and nine 1-gram packets of Sweet One® (approximately ⅓ cup).

When you use acesulfame potassium as a tabletop sweetener, such as Sweet One®, you aren't using it "neat." It is always mixed with one or more additional ingredients to reduce the level of sweetness to an equivalent of regular white granulated sugar (sucrose), to make sure it pours out of the packet easily, and to give it texture. If you check the ingredients label, for example, on the little 1-gram tabletop packet of Sweet One®, you will find it contains ▶**dextrose**, acesulfame potassium, cream of tartar, calcium silicate (an anticaking agent), and natural flavors.

▶ ACESULFAME POTASSIUM AT A GLANCE

Nonnutritive

Sweetness relative to sucrose About 200 times sweeter

Calories 0

FDA approval Yes

EFSA Number E950

ADI 15 mg (FDA and JECFA); 9 mg (EFSA) per kilogram (2.2 pounds) of body weight

ADVANTAME

About 20,000 times sweeter than regular white ▶**granulated sugar** (▶**sucrose**) and chemically related to ▶**aspartame**, advantame was developed by Ajinomoto Co., Inc. As a ▶**protein** it does provide 4 calories per gram, but the intensity of its sweetness means that such a minute amount is needed to achieve the desired sweetness, it is unlikely to add any calories overall in most foods and drinks or have any effect on ▶**blood glucose** levels; thus, it is considered a ▶**nonnutritive sweetener**.

Like aspartame and ▶**neotame**, it is partially absorbed in the small intestine and rapidly metabolized and excreted in urine and feces. Although it contains phenylalanine, such a minute amount of advantame is needed to sweeten foods that exposure to phenylalanine is insignificant. As a result, regulatory authorities such as the FDA and FSANZ do not require a label warning for people with phenylketonuria (PKU; see page 243). At the time of publication, no consumer products were available.

▶ ADVANTAME AT A GLANCE

Nonnutritive

Sweetness relative to sucrose About 20,000 times sweeter

Calories 0

FDA approval Yes

EFSA Number E969

ADI 5 mg (EFSA) per kilogram (2.2 pounds) of body weight

AGAVE NECTAR OR SYRUP

The first samples of this sweeter-than-▶**granulated sugar**, slightly runnier-than-▶**honey** syrup were introduced into the United States at Expo West in 1995 by Colibree's Sabra Van Dolsen and Humberto Saldana Pico. They had been specially manufactured at a pilot plant at the University of Guadalajara. It was perfect timing, tapping into a growing market of health-conscious consumers seeking natural options to regular granulated sugar and of vegans looking for alternatives to honey. Today, agave nectar is big business, and this alternative sweetener is found on the shelves of major supermarkets and small independent natural and ▶**organic** grocery stores worldwide.

The nectar is extracted from the sap of several species of agave, most famously blue agave (*Agave tequilana* F.A.C. Weber), Mexico's large (6 to 8 feet tall) and spiky succulent that also gives the world tequila. It typically takes about seven years for the sugar content in an agave plant's sap to peak (it needs to be at least 24 percent) and be ready for harvesting. The leaves are then cut away to reveal the fibrous *piña*, or heart, of the plant, which is crushed to extract the sap. The sap is immediately filtered and heated or treated enzymatically to convert its not-very-sweet ▶**fructans** (see the Buzz Notes on page 24) into the much-sweeter ▶**fructose** and ▶**glucose** (see ▶**carbohydrate** for more details). The amount of fructose can range from 55 to 90 percent depending on the variety of agave and the processing method. For example, tests by GI Labs in Toronto demonstrated that the amount of fructose in the iidea Company's brand of agave nectars ranged from 70 to 78 percent fructose for the light standard syrup to 78 to 85 percent for the light premium syrup (significantly more fructose than you find in ▶**high fructose corn syrup**).

The typically high fructose content of this sweetener gives it a low glycemic index range (GI 19 to 28), making it popular with people who have diabetes and must manage their ▶**blood glucose** levels. It has the same number of calories per level teaspoon as granulated sugar, but it is about 30 to 40 percent sweeter, so you can use less—just as well, because it generally costs more.

Like other syrups, there are several grades of agave nectar to choose from that vary in flavor, intensity, and color. As a rule of thumb, the neutral flavor of light agave nectar is best for sweetening beverages or replacing granulated sugar in recipes, and the more mellow flavors of amber, dark, or raw agave nectar are best for adding to tangy dressings, sauces, marinades, and glazes; drizzling over pancakes or oatmeal; or replacing light or dark ▶**brown sugar** in recipes. Agave nectar has also proved very popular with mixologists, because it can be used in almost any recipe that calls for ▶**simple syrup** and is a natural choice for tequila-based cocktails. The agave that bartenders use is a cocktail-ready, easy-to-pour syrup that can flow through pour spouts and not clog up in cocktail shakers.

When substituting it for sugar in a recipe, remember to allow for agave nectar's extra sweetness. Use two-thirds to three-quarters the amount of agave than the amount of ▶**granulated sugar** called for, and, in baking, reduce the liquid by about ¼ cup to adjust for the fact that you are adding moisture. You can substitute agave nectar for ▶**honey** or ▶**maple syrup** one-for-one, as it has approximately the same moisture content. However, if you want to use it in your cooking, we suggest you start with recipes that already list agave nectar in the ingredients. This way, you will become familiar with how much to use to achieve optimal sweetness, flavor, and texture before using it to replace honey or other sugars in your favorite recipes.

▶ AGAVE NECTAR OR SYRUP AT A GLANCE

Nutritive

Sugars Fructose, glucose

Sweetness relative to sucrose About 30–40% sweeter

Calories 21 calories (88 kilojoules) per level teaspoon

Health Contains ▶**FODMAPs**

I have heard agave has no carbs. Is that right?

This is a common misconception. Agave, like other sources of ▶**nutritive** sugars and ▶**sweeteners**, contains ▶**carbohydrates**. In fact, a level teaspoon of agave syrup or nectar contains just as many carbohydrates as does a level teaspoon of sugar. But as agave syrup is about 30 to 40 percent sweeter than sugar, in theory you need less.

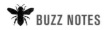 **BUZZ NOTES**
Fructans

You probably eat fructans more often than you realize. They are a type of dietary ▶**fiber** that occurs in plant foods such as agave, artichokes, asparagus, unripe bananas, carrots, ▶**chicory root**, garlic, Jerusalem artichokes, jicama, leeks, onions, wheat, and ▶**yacon syrup**. In simple terms, a fructan is a chain of ▶**fructose** molecules joined together. Short-chain fructans are known as ▶**fructooligosaccharides** and are about 30 percent as sweet as regular white ▶**granulated sugar** (▶**sucrose**); longer-chain fructans are known as ▶**inulins** and are only about 10 percent as sweet as granulated sugar.

AGAVE POWDER

(sweet agave powder)

Think of agave powder as sweet dietary ▶**fiber**. The term tends to be applied to three products: powdered ▶**fructose** with agave ▶**inulin**; 100 percent agave inulin; and agave inulin plus ▶**maltodextrin**. Agave powder's sweetness and fiber content will depend on the brand and the blend, so check the label or product information to be clear about what you are buying.

If you're looking for agave powder or agave inulin, you are more likely to find products online than on the shelves of your local supermarket or even health food store. Because the powder is highly soluble and its sweetness varies, check the label or manufacturer's website for substitution instructions before spooning it into the mixing bowl.

▶ **AGAVE POWDER AT A GLANCE**

Nutritive

Sugars Fructose (Switter brand powdered fructose with agave inulin)

Sweetness relative to sucrose About 30% sweeter

Calories 20 calories (84 kilojoules) per level teaspoon (Switter brand)

Health Contains ▶**FODMAPs**

ALITAME

(See page 270 for brand names)

About 2,000 times sweeter than regular white ▶**granulated sugar** (▶**sucrose**) and chemically related to ▶**aspartame**, this dipeptide is made up of two amino acids (L-aspartic acid and D-alanine amide). It was developed by Pfizer in the early 1980s. It is not literally a ▶**zero-calorie sweetener** (as a ▶**protein**, it does provide 4 calories per gram), but it is considered a ▶**nonnutritive sweetener** because the intensity of its sweetness means that such a minute amount is needed to achieve the desired sweetness, it adds only 1 to 2 calories overall in most foods and drinks and has no effect on ▶**blood glucose** levels. Between 7 to 22 percent of alitame passes through the body, is excreted in feces, and flushed away without being metabolized. Unlike aspartame, it does not contain phenylalanine; thus people with PKU (phenylketonuria; see page 243) can use it if they wish.

Alitame is heat stable and highly soluble in water and has a synergistic sweetening effect when combined with other intense sweeteners. It does not have FDA approval, so it can't be used in the United States; nor has it been approved in Canada. However, it is approved for use in Australia, China, Mexico, New Zealand, and the European Union for all food and beverage products, although it does not appear to be widely used in processed foods or beverages.

▶ **ALITAME AT A GLANCE**

Nonnutritive

Sweetness relative to sucrose About 2,000 times sweeter

Calories 0

FDA approval No

EFSA Number E956

ADI 1 mg (JECFA) per kilogram (2.2 pounds) of body weight

ARTIFICIAL SWEETENERS

(▶*nonnutritive sweeteners (NNS)*; ▶*high-intensity sweeteners (HIS); see page 270 for brand names*)

Artificial sweetener is a term used to differentiate the nonnutritive sugar alternatives created in a laboratory from their zero-calorie or low-calorie counterparts extracted from plant products such as a leaf

(▶**stevia**), a fruit (▶**monk fruit**), or a ▶**polyol** (▶**xylitol**). The distinction matters, because the sweetener industry itself sees those sugar-substitute compounds derived from plant (and microbial) extracts as a significant area of future growth and can (and already do) market them to consumers as "natural" sweeteners.

Most products labeled "diet" or "diabetic-friendly," including soft drinks, yogurts, candy, breath mints, and gum, contain artificial sweeteners in minute amounts. For example, a breath mint has around 1.5 milligrams ▶**aspartame**, a stick of gum 6 to 8 milligrams, an 8-ounce (200-gram) tub of yogurt around 124 milligrams, and a 12-ounce (350-milliliter) can of carbonated soft drink some 180 milligrams, according to the NutraSweet Company's website.

In consumer products, such as tabletop sweeteners, artificial sweeteners are not used solo. That virtually weightless sachet of Equal® Original (equivalent to 2 level teaspoons of sugar) you add to your tea or coffee contains ▶**dextrose** with ▶**maltodextrin**, aspartame, and ▶**acesulfame potassium** according to its US website, equal.com/equal-next/ingredients, at the time of writing.

Are they safe? There are many stories floating around on the Internet about this. The concern is not new—▶**saccharin**'s safety was first questioned when it was invented well over one hundred years ago. What we can say is that the sweeteners that have been approved for use as food additives (a long and rigorous process) by regulatory authorities such as the United States FDA have been studied more thoroughly than any other type of food additive. In approving these food additives, the regulatory bodies set rules as to how they may be used, as well as an Acceptable Daily Intake (ADI) based on body weight (see page 9 for a definition of ADI). For example, the FDA approved the use of acesulfame potassium in foods and as a tabletop sweetener in 1988, in beverages in 1998, and as a general-use sweetener in 2003. They set the ADI at 15 milligrams per kilogram (2.2 pounds) of body weight per day. The FDA keeps a register of any reported adverse effects, and, to date, no convincing evidence has been presented that the currently approved artificial sweeteners are harmful to health.

Are they for everyone? No. Although it is not known if they will affect the health of a rapidly developing fetus, many health professionals and medical organizations such as American Medical Association recommend that pregnant women avoid products containing the sweeteners saccharin and/or ▶**cyclamate,** because they can cross the placenta into the growing fetus and can also be found in breast milk. In addition, aspartame is not appropriate for anyone with the rare and serious condition PKU (phenylketonuria; see page 243).

How should you use them? Health authorities recommend that people who choose to use ▶**zero-calorie sweeteners** (or diet products that include them) opt for a variety of nonnutritive sweeteners to reduce the likelihood of excessive consumption of any single one.

The pros and cons? These nonnutritive sweeteners have virtually no effect on ▶**blood glucose** levels and can help you cut back on your calories if you use them to replace equivalent amounts of sugar or ▶**honey**, etc. Their major drawback is that they aren't as versatile as sugar and honey and other ▶**nutritive sweeteners**. This is because they don't tend to be heat stable or to brown, caramelize, and add texture or bulk to food when used in baking. They also tend to be much more expensive, gram for gram, than their nutritive sweetener counterparts.

Do they actually do their job and help with weight loss? "It is not uncommon for people to be given messages that artificially sweetened products are healthy, will help them lose weight, or will help prevent weight gain," says Susan E. Swithers, PhD, of Purdue University, in a press release.[7] "The data to support those claims are not very strong, and although it seems like common sense that diet sodas would not be as problematic as regular sodas, common sense is not always right." Aspartame and ▶**sucralose**, for example, were introduced into the Australian food supply in the early 1980s and 1990s, respectively, and since then sugar consumption has been reduced by about 10 percent, suggesting that Australians have been using them instead of regular ▶**granulated sugar (sucrose)**. However, since the early 1980s, rates of overweight and obesity have nearly doubled in Australia. Similar trends have been reported in studies of nonnutritive sweetener consumption in the United States.[8] So, there are real questions to be asked:

- Do people overcompensate when they consume nonnutritive sweeteners by eating more high-calorie foods—for example, digging in to a hamburger with the works and large fries when they buy a diet soft drink?
- Do nonnutritive sweeteners have a negative effect on the bacteria in our guts (our microbiome), predisposing some people to weight gain?

- Do people mistakenly assume that foods sweetened with nonnutritive sweeteners are calorie-free and therefore over-eat them?
- Do nonnutritive sweeteners confuse the way our brain regulates our feelings of hunger and fullness?

We believe that much more research is needed to answer this question. Perhaps it is a bit of all four? *See also* ▶**acesulfame K**; ▶**alitame**; ▶**aspartame**; ▶**cyclamate**; ▶**neotame**; ▶**nonnutritive sweeteners**; ▶**saccharin**; ▶**sucralose**; ▶**thaumatin**

ASPARTAME

(See page 270 for brand names)

Aspartame is one of the most tested food additives in FDA history and is currently found in over six thousand foods and beverages, including Coca-Cola and Pepsi products. It all started with a lucky lab accident. Back in 1965, when James Schlatter was developing a peptic-ulcer drug for the pharmaceutical company G. D. Searle, he licked his finger and found that the powdery substance he was working on was surprisingly sweet. (As it turns out, it is around 200 times sweeter on average than regular ▶**granulated sugar/sucrose**.) Since achieving FDA approval in 1981, aspartame has been the ▶**artificial sweetener** at the forefront of the worldwide explosion of zero-calorie and low-calorie foods and beverages.

In the body, aspartame breaks down during digestion into aspartic acid and phenylalanine, which are both amino acids (the building blocks from which all proteins are made), as well as a small amount of methanol, a substance naturally found in foods such as meat, milk, fruits, and vegetables. It is generally regarded as safe by the FDA and food authorities around the world except for anyone with PKU (phenylketonuria; see page 243). Aspartame contains a significant amount of phenylalanine, which people with PKU should avoid. This is why the warning "Contains phenylalanine" appears on all aspartame-based tabletop sweeteners and foods and beverages sweetened with aspartame.

Because it is chemically a ▶**protein**, it is not literally a ▶**zero-calorie sweetener**, since all proteins provide 4 calories per gram. However, the intensity of aspartame's sweetness means that such minute amounts are needed that it adds only 1 to 2 calories overall in most foods and drinks and has no effect on ▶**blood glucose** levels. For example, if you downed a 12-ounce (350-milliliter) diet soda containing 125 milligrams of aspartame, you would add less than 1 calorie to your diet. The same-sized soda sweetened with sugar would add around 140 calories (600 kilojoules).

Different brands offer a variety of aspartame sweetener products for different uses, so it is hard to generalize about what's in them and how to use them. However, manufacturers of the "spoon-for-spoon" granulated-sugar substitutes typically add ▶**maltodextrin** as a bulking agent. For example, the ingredients listed for Equal Spoonful are maltodextrin, aspartame, and ▶**acesulfame potassium** (often blended with aspartame). If you want to cook with an aspartame-based product, check the manufacturer's website for substitution tips. *See also* ▶**nonnutritive sweeteners**

▶ **ASPARTAME AT A GLANCE**
Nonnutritive
Sweetness relative to sucrose About 150–250 times sweeter
Calories 0
FDA approval Yes
EFSA Number E951
ADI 50 mg (FDA); 40 mg (EFSA and JECFA) per kilogram (2.2 pounds) of body weight

BAKER'S SUGAR OR BAKER'S SPECIAL

This is a professional grade of ▶**superfine sugar** (▶**sucrose**) used by bakers. Its fine crystal dissolves, mixes, blends, and melts very evenly, producing an end product with a fine, delicate crumb.

BAR SUGAR

The "bars" we are talking about here are cocktail bars, not solid blocks. This is another name for ▶**superfine sugar** (▶**sucrose**), coined because bartenders appreciate how easily the ultrafine crystals dissolve in mixed drinks and in making a ▶**simple syrup**.

BARBADOS SUGAR

The ▶**muscovado sugar** shipped from Barbados to refineries in Britain during the seventeenth, eighteenth, and nineteenth centuries was (and sometimes still is) known as Barbados sugar. It is partially refined ▶**cane sugar** (▶**sucrose**) with a distinctive aroma and ▶**molasses** flavor. You may see it described on packaging as "unrefined." Light and dark muscovado (Barbados) sugars are available. Both are interchangeable with regular ▶**brown sugar** in recipes.

BARLEY MALT

(barley malt extract, barley malt syrup, barley syrup, malt extract, malt syrup)

It's the barley malt that makes the difference. Without it, a traditional New York City bagel—which otherwise consists of flour, yeast, water, egg, and salt—would be just a chewy roll with a hole. Barley malt also makes a difference in many other foods and beverages: breads (especially rye and whole grain breads), breakfast cereals, cookies, candy (think malted milk balls), and milk flavoring products such as Ovaltine®, Horlicks®, and Milo®.

The barley malt story, which goes back thousands of years to the time when our hunter-gatherer forebears first settled down, begins with brewing. Ancient pottery jars dating back some seven thousand years in Mesopotamia (the area of the Tigris–Euphrates river system) provide us with telltale signs of beer-barley fermentation, while a song of praise to the Sumerian goddess of brewing, Ninkasi ("who soaks the malt in the jar"), gives us the first written recipe for malting and beer making.

These days we tend to think of barley simply as that slow-cooking, starchy grain you can add to vegetable soups or use in a different spin on risottos. But beer lovers know that good beer begins with barley, because it's the grain best suited for malting, a process that converts the starch in the grain into the sugar ►**maltose**, which contributes to the beer's color, flavor, sweetness, body, foam, and mouthfeel. If the liquid extracted from the mashing process of the wort (meaning, plant, pronounced "wirt") is not fermented but instead evaporated, the result is barley malt, a rich brown syrupy extract that's about half as sweet as ►**sucrose** with a distinctive flavor and a consistency similar to that of ►**molasses** or ►**golden syrup**. Because it is barley-based, this sweetener is not suitable for anyone on a gluten-free diet. Its glycemic index has not been tested, but as a malted syrup, it will have a very high glycemic index. We estimate it is up there with ►**rice syrup** (GI 98), as the sugars it contains are the same: maltose, ►**maltotriose**, and ►**glucose**.

Although not as popular as rice syrup, ►**maple syrup**, or ►**honey**, barley malt is a versatile sweetener. You can drizzle it over cereals and pancakes or brush it onto sweet potatoes and winter squash or meats as a glaze before roasting them. In baking, it is best suited to recipes that call for ►**brown sugar**, such as muffins and quick breads with dried fruit, gingerbread, spice cakes, and darker, whole-grain breads. When substituting it for ►**granulated sugar** or honey, remember that barley malt is only about half as sweet, so you need to use more, which will mean more calories. Generally it's recommended to replace 1 cup of sugar with 1⅓ cups of barley malt and reduce the liquid in the recipe by about ¼ cup, but be guided by the texture of the batter or dough.

You may also see a suggestion to take a spoonful of barley malt extract "as part of a balanced diet and healthy lifestyle," which might seem odd in these sugar-wary times. It is a reminder, however, that throughout the first half of the twentieth century, malt extract was very much seen as a restorative that could put color into children's cheeks and, combined with cod liver oil, help build strong bones (i.e., prevent rickets). Indeed, Kanga gives a reluctant Roo and an enthusiastic Tigger a strengthening dose of malt extract in *The House at Pooh Corner*, and the Pabst Brewing Company, today best known for its Blue Ribbon lager, once advertised its malt extract as a way to "keep strong always" and "make every atom of your vitality count." If this makes you feel nostalgic, you can buy malt extract with cod liver oil in three flavors (butterscotch, honey, and natural) from the British company Potter's Herbals, which has relaunched its original malt extract. *See also* ▶**malt**

▶ **BARLEY MALT AT A GLANCE**
   Nutritive
   Sugars Maltose, maltotriose, glucose
   Sweetness relative to sucrose About 50% as sweet
   Calories 16 calories (67 kilojoules) per level teaspoon (USDA: "Malt syrup")
   Health Contains gluten

 Why is barley malt used in bread recipes?

Bread bakers like to use malt because it not only contributes flavor and color, but also does not interfere with gluten development (▶**sucrose** does), and because it is a diastatic malt and therefore contains enzymes that convert flour (▶**starch)** to sugar (yeast food). ("Diastatic" refers to enzymes that convert starch to sugar and are created as the grain sprouts.)

BEET SUGAR

   See ▶*granulated sugar;* ▶*sucrose;* ▶*sugar beet*

BERRY SUGAR

You may occasionally find this listed in the ingredients for baking shortbread or meringues, especially in older British recipes. It is just another name for ▶**superfine sugar**. We have tracked down one brand still on the market: Roger's Berry Sugar in Canada.

BIRCH SUGAR

Derived from birch bark, birch sugar (▶**xylitol**) was first used as a sweetener in Finland during World War II, when regular sugar was unavailable. It is a ▶**polyol (sugar alcohol)** that occurs naturally in the fibers of many fruits and vegetables but is today extracted commercially from various hardwoods and corncobs.

BIRCH SYRUP

People have been tapping birch trees for centuries in the taiga of Europe and Asia to enjoy the therapeutic benefits of the refreshing sap that tastes like slightly sweet water. They also used it to make syrup, wine, beer, and vinegars to stock their pantries for the rest of the year. Today, most of the world's commercially produced birch syrup comes from North America and principally Alaska, even though serious production only began there in the late 1980s.

Like ▶**maple syrup**, it is made by collecting sap (in this case from birch trees) and reducing it down to a syrup that is about 60 to 70 percent sugar. But there are some extra production challenges, because birch sap is very different chemically from maple sap. First, it typically contains around 1 percent sugar, so producers need 80 to 100 gallons of sap to make 1 gallon of syrup. (Maple sap is around 2 percent sugar, so producers need only about 40 to 50 gallons of sap for that gallon of syrup—half the amount needed for birch syrup.) Second, birch syrup makers can't simply boil down the sap as maple sugar makers do. They need to distill it at a lower temperature, because birch sap's main sugar is ▶**fructose**, which burns or scorches at a much lower temperature than does ▶**sucrose**, maple sap's main sugar.

The final product is about one-third water and two-thirds sugars, consisting of about 42 to 54 percent fructose and 45 percent ▶**glucose**, with a small amount of sucrose and trace amounts of ▶**galactose**. Its glycemic index has not been tested, but we estimate that it is low.

Currently birch syrup is more gourmet market than mass market; it is typically three to five times more expensive than maple syrup, thanks to its production challenges, transport costs, limited supply, and growing demand. It has a distinctive flavor that many cooks find best suited to marinades, barbecue sauces, glazes, and dressings. In Alaska, it is also used to make a variety of specialty "birch syrup" flavored food products such as candy, baked goods, condiments, and ice cream. Sweeter birch syrup blends with added fructose or maple syrup are also available and tend to be a better choice for drizzling over pancakes or waffles.

▶ **BIRCH SYRUP AT A GLANCE**
Nutritive
Sugars Fructose, glucose, sucrose, galactose
Sweetness relative to sucrose Equally sweet
Calories 16 calories (67 kilojoules) per level teaspoon
Health Contains ▶FODMAPs

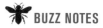 **BUZZ NOTES**
Birch Water

Straight from the tree, birch sap was a traditional springtime tonic in northern Europe, known as birch water and renowned for its strengthening and curative powers. Over two hundred years ago, Baron Pierre-François Percy, army surgeon and inspector general to Napoleon, extolled its benefits: "Throughout the whole of northern Europe . . . birch water is the hope, the blessing, and the panacea of rich and poor, master and peasant alike . . . It almost unfailingly cures skin conditions such as pimples, scurf, acne, etc., it is an invaluable remedy for rheumatic diseases, the after-effects of gout, bladder obstructions, and countless chronic ills against which medical science is so prone to fail." These days, it's not just a springtime beverage. It is bottled and sold as a refreshing health drink with 1 to 1½ percent natural sugars in Japan, Korea, Scandinavia, and Eastern Europe. Leading brands include Denmark's Sealand Birk and Finland's Nordic Koivu.

BLACKSTRAP MOLASSES

This thick, dark syrup is powerful stuff best kept for robust recipes that actually call for it in the list of ingredients. With a hearty, slightly bitter flavor, blackstrap molasses is not a suitable substitute in cooking and baking for the sweeter and milder light and dark molasses products. While all ►**molasses** is a by-product of the various centrifugal stages of ►**cane sugar** refining, blackstrap (from the Dutch *stroop*, meaning, "syrup") comes from the third and final spinning and is the most concentrated, least sweet, and darkest in color.

BLACK SUGAR

(►*Japanese black sugar*, ►*kokuto*, ►*Okinawan black sugar/ brown sugar*)

►**Sugarcane** has been grown in Okinawa since the seventeenth century. The traditional black sugar made from it isn't actually black; it is a very dark brown, partially refined sugar similar to ►**jaggery**. Today, it is still made by slowly cooking down the cane juice very much the way it was done hundreds of years ago. After the cane stalks are crushed to release their juice, the juice is boiled in open pans to evaporate most of the water. The concentrated, thick syrup is then transferred to other pans, stirred, and left to cool and set, producing a solid piece of ►**sucrose** that is then chopped into pieces. In larger operations, the finished sugar may be spun in a centrifuge to cool it and remove moisture. It has not been glycemic index tested, but as it is sucrose, we estimate it has a moderate glycemic index.

Black sugar is a key ingredient in many traditional Okinawan dishes, such as stir-fries, stews, soups, and salads. You can find it in specialty Japanese or Asian produce stores or online. Alternatively, replace it in recipes with other partially refined ►**cane sugars** such as ►**muscovado** or ►**panela**, or regular moist dark ►**brown sugar**.

► **BLACK SUGAR AT A GLANCE**

Nutritive

Sugars Sucrose

Sweetness relative to sucrose Equally sweet

Calories 16 calories (67 kilojoules) per level teaspoon

BLACK TREACLE

Thick, black, and "gloopy," this is a British classic still sold in its classic tin. A by-product of the sugar (►**sucrose**) refining process, black treacle adds color, moisture, and a rich molasses flavor to traditional British recipes such as gingerbread, Christmas pudding, parkin (a soft oatmeal cake), and treacle tart. It can also be used in glazes, barbecue sauce, and home brewing. Lyle's, a popular brand, is now available worldwide, but you can also substitute ▶**molasses**. *See also* ▶**treacle**

BLOOD GLUCOSE

Blood glucose, popularly called blood sugar, is the ▶**glucose** that travels through our bloodstream, supplying energy to all the cells in the body and brain. We can't live without it; we certainly can't think without it. When we consume foods that contain ▶**carbohydrates** (sugars and ▶**starches**), such as breads, breakfast cereals, rice, noodles, and pasta; fruits and berries; starchy vegetables such as potatoes and legumes; and milk and yogurt, our bodies convert the carbohydrates during digestion and metabolism to glucose (or blood glucose), which circulates in our bloodstream and is the universal fuel for our body's cells; the only fuel source for our brain, red blood cells, and a growing fetus; and the main source of energy for our muscles during strenuous exercise—just ask any athlete. We explain this in more detail in Health Matters (Sugars, Sweeteners, and Digestion, page 221).

BRAZZEIN

This naturally sweet ▶**protein** was isolated from the fruit of *Penta-diplandra brazzeana*, a shrub or vine growing in West Africa from Nigeria east to the Central African Republic and south to the Democratic Republic of Congo and Angola. The sweetness of the fruit is legendary among the locals, who enjoy it as a snack or use its delicious red pulp to sweeten their corn porridge. The story behind the fruit's alternative name, ▶**oubli** (French for "forget"), popular in parts of West Africa, is that small children who eat the supersweet berries get so distracted that they completely forget to return home—like any kid in a candy store.

Brazzein is reported to be between 500 and 2,000 times sweeter than sugar (▶**sucrose**), and a ▶**zero-calorie sweetener** (Cweet®) is being developed based on it. The brazzein protein in Cweet is not extracted from the fruit but is synthesized using a special process patented by the University of Wisconsin, Madison. At the time of publication, Cweet has not been approved for use in foods or beverages by any food authority. *See also* ▶**proteins, sweet-tasting**

BREWING SUGARS AND SYRUPS

Beer making may begin with ▶**malt**, but ▶**maltose** is not the only sugar involved in the brew. Other sugars and syrups, used in smaller quantities, impart distinctive characteristics to a beer, setting apart a stout, for example, from a porter. Sugars and syrups can also increase the strength of a beer without substantially increasing its body or changing its flavor profile, as well as prime a beer for carbonation. ▶**Corn sugar** (▶**glucose**), which is often labeled "▶**dextrose**" on the package in a home brew kit, is the most common refined sugar used in home brewing. It is popular because it tends to be more fermentable and leaves a cleaner, crisper aftertaste than regular white ▶**granulated sugar** (▶**sucrose**). A product labeled "brewing sugar" may be 100 percent dextrose or a dextrose/▶**maltodextrin** mix, so check the ingredients label. Cooper's Brewing Sugar, for example, is 80 percent dextrose and 20 percent maltodextrin. Many brewing products are made from sucrose. The renowned Belgian ▶**candi sugar** (or syrup) is an ▶**invert sugar**—its sucrose has been broken down into glucose and ▶**fructose**.

For guidance on adding sugars and syrups to beer for flavor, we turned to a serious home brewer. John Palmer, author of the definitive *How to Brew: Everything You Need to Know to Brew Beer Right the First Time*, says:

> Various sugars have various flavors. The monosaccharides do not have a definable flavor other than sweet. But other sugars like honey, maple syrup, and molasses have characteristic flavors that can make a nice accent for a beer. This is what home brewing is all about, really—taking a standard beer style and dressing it up for your own tastes. You can make a maple syrup porter, or a honey raspberry wheat, or an imperial Russian stout with hints of rum and treacle. The possibilities are myriad. On the other hand, I have coined a phrase that will serve you well in your experimentation, "The better part of

flavor is discretion." A beer with 20 percent molasses is going to taste like fermented molasses, not beer.

Check out John's book for more expert home-brewing information, delivered with wit and wisdom.

BROWN RICE SYRUP

(▶ rice syrup, rice malt syrup)

This mild-flavored sweetener dissolves easily and is used in drinks, dressings, and baking and as a topping for cereals, waffles, and pancakes. It is popular with people who need (or want) to avoid ▶**fructose** and with those adopting a so-called "sugar-free" diet. We say "so-called" because brown rice syrup is not sugar-free. As a malted grain sweetener, it contains ▶**maltose**, ▶**maltotriose**, and ▶**glucose**—all types of sugar. Nor is it low glycemic or "slow digesting," as some manufacturers claim on their websites and labels. The University of Sydney GI database (glycemicindex.com) lists the glycemic index as GI 98—that's really very high. If you are substituting rice syrup for ▶**granulated sugar** (sucrose) in a recipe, you will need to use more to achieve the equivalent level of sweetness, which also means more calories—and a greater glycemic impact (glycemic load).

Tip: Don't assume it is gluten-free because it is a rice-based food product. Check the label, as some producers use barley enzymes in the malting process.

▶ BROWN RICE SYRUP AT A GLANCE
Nutritive
Sugars Maltose, glucose, maltotriose
Sweetness relative to sucrose About 70% as sweet
Calories 16 calories (67 kilojoules) per level teaspoon
Health May contain gluten

BROWN SUGAR, SOFT

(light brown sugar, golden brown sugar, golden yellow sugar)

There's nothing quite like a spoonful of soft brown sugar sprinkled on oatmeal. Moist, dark, and slightly clumpy, it melts over the surface and transforms a traditional hot cereal into a sweet treat to fuel your day.

THE ULTIMATE GUIDE TO SUGARS & SWEETENERS

Generally speaking, the regular soft brown sugars you find in the supermarket are not naturally brown. They are blends: white ▶**granulated sugar** with a thin coating of ▶**molasses** syrup sprayed on. They vary in flavor and color from light and mild to dark and strong. Light brown (sometimes called yellow, light yellow, golden yellow, or brilliant yellow) sugar contains 3.5 percent molasses; dark, 6.5 percent. It's the naturally hygroscopic (moisture-retaining) molasses that gives these sugars their moist, clumping tendency. It is a good idea to keep soft brown sugar in an airtight container in a cool, dry place (or the freezer) once you have opened the package; otherwise it can dry out and go lumpy. To resoften, cooking guru Harold McGee suggests heating lumps in the microwave for 20 to 30 seconds or sealing them in a plastic bag with a piece of apple or fresh bread for a few hours.

You may sometimes hear that brown sugars are more healthful than white. However, although the molasses may contribute vitamins and minerals not found in white sugar, the amounts are too minute to count toward your recommended daily intake in an appreciable way. It still has all the calories that regular sugar has, and, as a pure ▶**sucrose** product, it has a moderate glycemic index (GI 65).

Remember: sugar is not a health food, and it never will be. But brown sugar can boost flavor or make some really healthy foods more palatable. Used this way, a little brown sugar can go a long way: sprinkle it over ripe Roma tomato halves before roasting them; create a balanced Asian salad dressing with lime juice, fish sauce, and brown sugar; or caramelize 3 to 4 tablespoons of balsamic vinegar with 1 tablespoon of brown sugar and drizzle it over crispy baked sweet potatoes.

Many home bakers opt for brown sugar. It is especially suited to cookies, cereal bars, gingerbread, muffins, carrot cakes, fruitcakes, and Christmas mince pies because it retains moisture better than granulated white sugar does. In savory foods, brown sugar is an ideal addition to condiments and glazes for meats and vegetables, and its rich, full flavor makes homemade baked beans shine. You can substitute soft brown sugar for granulated white sugar cup for cup. Because the white sugar is denser than the brown, you need to firmly pack brown sugar into the measuring cup to get a level measure and equal sweetness.

What about blends? Increasingly, blends of regular sugar (brown and white) with a ▶**nonnutritive sweetener**, especially ▶**stevia**, are available. They will save you calories. However, if you want to use them in your baking, we suggest you first try one of the manufacturer's tested recipes before substituting for regular sugar in your own recipes. It is also worth checking the ingredient list. You need to be aware that some blends, such as Truvia® Brown Sugar Blend, include ▶**erythritol** (a ▶**polyol**) as well as brown sugar and stevia.

▶ SOFT BROWN SUGAR AT A GLANCE

Nutritive

Sugars Sucrose

Sweetness relative to sucrose Equally sweet

Calories 16 calories (67 kilojoules) per level teaspoon

Sweet records

TEXAS: On November 30, 2013, the World's Largest Gingerbread House was built out of 1,800 pounds of butter, 7,200 eggs, 7,200 pounds of flour, and close to 3,000 pounds of brown sugar. Add in the 22,304 pieces of candy attached to it, and the calorie count grand total came to 35,823,400 calories! No one nibbled the 60-by-42-feet gingerbread house. It was a fund-raiser and was "deconstructed" a couple of weeks later. (Traditions Golf Club partnered with the St. Joseph Health System and Thrive Home Health Care and donated all profits to St. Joseph's Level II Trauma Center.)

BULK SWEETENERS

(▶*polyols;* ▶*sugar alcohols*)

Polyols (sugar alcohols) are also known as bulk sweeteners, because they are essentially sweet "fillers" and generally can be used as a ▶**granulated sugar** substitute on a spoon-for-spoon basis. ▶**Erythritol**, ▶**isomalt**, ▶**lacititol**, ▶**maltitol**, ▶**mannitol**, ▶**sorbitol**, and ▶**xylitol** are all bulk sweeteners permitted for use in foods. They are mostly used by the food industry in desserts, ice cream, jam, preserves, baked goods, breakfast cereals, and sauces, for example, but you can buy some of them for personal use on their own or as part of a blend with a more intense sweetener such as ▶**monk fruit** or ▶**stevia**.

CANDI SUGAR

The renowned Belgian candi sugar (or syrup) is an ▶**invert sugar**—its ▶**sucrose** has been broken down into ▶**glucose** and ▶**fructose**. It is used as a ▶**brewing sugar**, especially in making stronger beers, as it boosts alcohol content without adding extra body. It is also used as a ▶**priming sugar**.

CANE JUICE

▶**Sugarcane**, with its 16 to 18 percent ▶**sucrose**-rich juice, has long been prized for its sweetness. In cane-growing countries, street vendors and their sugarcane-juice carts are a familiar sight, and the juice is also popping up in stalls at trendy farmers' market stalls. An 8-ounce glass of sugarcane juice (250 milliliters or 1 cup) provides around 100 calories (420 kilojoules) and 20 grams of carbohydrates, close to a same-sized glass of apple juice with 108 calories (450 kilojoules) and 26 grams of carbohydrates. Sugarcane juice hasn't been glycemic index tested, but, given that it is sucrose and water, we would estimate it has a moderate glycemic index of around 65.

🐝 BUZZ NOTES

A study published in the *Asian Journal of Sports Medicine* in 2013 reports that cane juice appears to be as effective during exercise as either sports drinks or plain water (when environmental temperature is below 30°C/86°F) and more effective for rehydrating post-exercise, as it enhances muscle glycogen resynthesis (see page 77 for more on glycogen).[9]

CANE SUGAR

Sugar is one of the world's leading internationally traded commodities, with an annual value exceeding US $24 billion (2012). Around three-quarters of the world's sugar is made from ▶**sugarcane**, a perennial grass (*Saccharum officinarum*). The balance is from ▶**sugar beet**.

CANE SYRUP

Deep golden cane syrup with a sweeter-than-▶**molasses**, caramellike flavor is a feature of much southern United States and Caribbean cooking. It was traditionally made in open kettles, where the fresh juice extracted from the crushed cane stalks was slowly boiled down to the right consistency over several hours, during which time some of the ▶**sucrose** would invert (break down into separate ▶**glucose** and ▶**fructose** molecules). These days, producing cane syrup is essentially a cottage industry.

Cane syrup is available mainly in the southern United States or online. Drizzle it over pancakes or waffles or use it in gingerbread, pecan pie, baked beans, a glaze for baked ham, and other traditional Southern fare such as *gâteau de sirop* ("syrup cake") or shoofly pie. You can also substitute it for ▶**simple syrup** (AKA sugar syrup) in cocktails and mocktails.

▶ CANE SYRUP AT A GLANCE

Nutritive

Sugars Sucrose, glucose, fructose

Sweetness relative to sucrose Equally sweet

Calories 16 calories (67 kilojoules) per level teaspoon

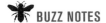 BUZZ NOTES
A Southern Icon

One of the few remaining producers of traditional Southern cane syrup, Steen's, of Abbeville, Louisiana, was recognized by the Slow Food Foundation for Biodiversity, which has added Steen's 100% Pure Cane Syrup to its "Ark of Taste." Like so much in the history of sugar and sweeteners, Steen's cane-syrup business happened by chance. In 1910, an early freeze hit Charley Steen Jr.'s cane crop. To save the day, Charley harvested and peeled the sugarcane, smashed the sweet pulp into juice (using horse-powered rollers back then), and boiled the juice down. The result? Steen's 100% Pure Cane Syrup.

CARBOHYDRATE

The term *carbohydrate* comes from chemistry and means "watered carbon" (carbon with water molecules). For example, the formula for glucose is C_6H12O_6 (six carbon atoms and six water molecules—$H2O$ = water). Sometimes you will see carbohydrate shortened to CHO, which stands for carbon, hydrogen, and oxygen.

One way to think of carbohydrates is as the life force of plants. This is because it is a vital source of energy found in all plants and in the foods we harvest from them. The simplest form of carbohydrate is a sweet-tasting, single-sugar molecule called a ▶**monosaccharide**. *Mono* means "one"; *saccharide* comes from the Latin *saccharum* (from the Greek *sakcharon*, and the Sanskrit *śarkarā*), which means "sugar." There are three common dietary monosaccharides, two of which come from plants (words ending in *-ose* are sugars):

> ▶**Fructose** is found in fruits, honey, and agave sap.
> ▶**Galactose** is found in milk, yogurt, and whey.
> ▶**Glucose** is found in fruits, grains, vegetables, and honey.

Two single-sugar molecules joined together is called a ▶**disaccharide** (*di* means "two"). Of three common sweet-tasting dietary disaccharides, two come from plants:

> ▶**Lactose**, which is glucose joined with galactose, is found in milk and yogurt. It has a low glycemic index (GI 46).
> ▶**Maltose**, which is two glucose molecules joined together, is found in grains such as barley and in malt and malted foods and beverages. It has a high glycemic index (GI 105).
> ▶**Sucrose**, which is glucose joined with fructose, is found in tubers such as potatoes, ▶**sugar beet**, the grass ▶**sugarcane**, the sap of ▶**maple** trees, and fruits. It has a moderate glycemic index (average GI 65).

Chains of three to nine single-sugar molecules are called ▶**oligosaccharides** (*oligo* means "a few"). They are only a little bit sweet. There are two classes of oligosaccharide used for sweetening:

▶**Fructooligosaccharides**, which are short chains of fructose molecules, are found in fruits and vegetables such as asparagus, bananas, ▶**chicory root**, garlic, Jerusalem artichokes, leeks, onions, wheat, and ▶**yacon**.

▶**Maltodextrins** (modified food ▶**starches**) are chains of glucose molecules ranging from three to nine glucose units long (think of them as a family of ingredients, not an individual one). They are produced by processing a starchy food such as corn, potatoes, rice, wheat, or tapioca to break down the starch. They are commonly used as food additives to provide bulk and texture, because they are only moderately sweet or even flavorless. You will also find them used as ingredients in single-serving tabletop packets of certain ▶**artificial sweeteners** and in pharmaceuticals. The FDA's Code of Federal Regulations (CFR) lists maltodextrin as a GRAS (Generally Recognized As Safe) additive.

Starches are ▶**polysaccharides** (*poly* means "many")—long chains (some branching, some straight) of single-sugar molecules. Starches are not sweet at all, but they can be broken down through a series of enzymatic conversions to provide us with glucose and maltose sweeteners such as ▶**barley malt**, ▶**corn syrup**, ▶**oat syrup**, ▶**rice syrup**, ▶**tapioca syrup**, ▶**wheat syrup**, etc.

Dietary ▶**fibers** are large carbohydrate molecules containing many different sorts of monosaccharides. Unlike starches and sugars, they are not broken down during digestion.

They come mostly (but not exclusively) from plants, and they are the poorly digested portions that pass through into the large intestine (bowel) and provide much of the bulk in our stool (along with water and bacteria, among a few other things). There are a number of ways of classifying the different types of fiber. One of the most popular systems is whether they are soluble in water or not:

- Water-soluble fibers include gums (e.g., agar), ▶**fructans** (e.g., ▶**inulin**), mucilages (e.g., psyllium), and pectins. They are found in a range of foods, including fruits, vegetables, legumes (beans, peas, and lentils), and some grains (oats and barley). Water-insoluble fibers include cellulose, hemicellulose, and lignin. They are mostly found in vegetables, wheat and other whole grains, nuts, and seeds.

The different types of dietary fibers have different effects on our health.

- Soluble dietary fiber may help reduce blood cholesterol levels and modulate ▶**blood glucose** levels—but whether it does so or not depends in part on the degree of food processing and, of course, on how much of it you eat. High cholesterol and blood glucose levels are risk factors for heart and other blood vessel diseases and type 2 diabetes, and there is evidence that high-fiber diets may help reduce the risk of heart disease and type 2 diabetes.
- Insoluble dietary fiber primarily helps with laxation, which in turn may decrease the risk of constipation, hemorrhoids, and colorectal (bowel) cancer.

Most of us need to eat more fiber—soluble and insoluble.

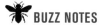 **BUZZ NOTES**
How Plants Make Sugars

All green plants make sugars by a process called photosynthesis, which you probably learned about in school. (Oxygen, you may recall, is a by-product of the process.) As a reminder, here's how it works: Plants draw water and minerals up from the soil through their roots and absorb carbon dioxide through their leaves. The green chlorophyll in the leaves then uses the sun's energy (sunlight) to combine the carbon dioxide and water and produce sugars—▶glucose, ▶fructose, and ▶sucrose. The sugars:

- Provide an immediate source of energy so plants can grow
- Provide an energy reserve, stored as sucrose, to keep plants growing when there's no sunlight or photosynthesis (e.g., nighttime)
- Are the building blocks for other substances plants need for growth and repair, such as cellulose (dietary fiber), which forms cell walls and provides structure and support
- Produce ▶**starch** (from glucose), which plants such as potatoes and rice store as an energy source.

How much carbohydrate should you eat?

▶**Carbohydrates** are an important part of your diet: they help keep your body sensitive to insulin, give you energy to think and do things, and provide stamina. Dietary guidelines from around the globe recommend that people eat between 45 to 60 percent of total calories (energy) from carbohydrates.

Dietary tools for people with diabetes focus on carbohydrates because they are the only part of food that directly affect ▶**blood glucose** levels. When we eat carbohydrate-containing foods, they are broken down into ▶**glucose**, and this raises our blood glucose levels. The body responds by releasing insulin into the blood. The insulin helps move glucose from the blood into your muscles and other organs, where it is used for energy, so the blood glucose level returns to normal. In people with diabetes, too many carbohydrates may result in high blood glucose levels (see page 221 for more on why this is, and page 231 for information on "carbohydrate exchanges").

What's a "low-carb" diet?

Low-carbohydrate diets are either high protein or high fat or both. They cannot be anything else, because you have to get your energy from something (and large amounts of alcohol, the only other energy source for humans, won't keep you alive for long). There are numerous variations of carbohydrate intake on a low-carb diet. There are low and very low options.

People who follow a typical "low-carb" diet will restrict their carbohydrates to around 80 to 130 grams a day of available (net) carbohydrates. People who follow a typical "very low-carb" or "ketogenic diet" will restrict their carbohydrates to around 20 to 50 grams a day of available (net) carbohydrates.

Consuming around 80 grams of available (net) carbohydrates a day might look like this: 1 medium apple; 1 cup orange juice; ½ cup oatmeal (porridge), 1 slice whole wheat bread, 1 small container (5 ounces/150 grams) fat-free, flavored Greek yogurt, 1 cup reduced-fat milk.

Consuming around 20 to 30 grams of available (net) carbohydrates a day might look like this: 1 medium apple, ⅔ cup reduced-fat milk.

The "ketogenic" variation is often found in the "kick-start" phase of popular diet books. It is not recommended for women who are pregnant or breastfeeding.

Some problems you can experience if you don't have enough carbohydrates in your diet:

- Muscle fatigue, causing moderate exercise to cost an enormous effort
- Insufficient fiber intake, causing constipation
- Headaches and tiredness due to low blood glucose levels
- Bad breath due to the breakdown products of fat (ketones).

What's the difference between available (net) carbs and total carbs?

This seemingly simple question is complicated for several reasons including the labeling regulations of the country you live in. In the United States, for example, the total carbohydrate (in grams) listed on the nutrition facts panel *includes* fiber. In many other parts of the world, including Australia and New Zealand, the total carbohydrate listed in the nutrition information panel *excludes* ▶**fiber**, which, unlike ▶**starches** and sugars, is not broken down during digestion. In these countries, the resulting carbohydrate count is sometimes referred to as "available" or "net" carbs. Many low-carb weight-loss plans, including the new Atkins diet, also use "net carbs" in their diet plans.

We have put together the following table of some healthy, carb-rich foods using the US diabetes exchange tables for "total carbs" and Australia's food tables for available or "net" carbs to give you an idea of the difference in the numbers. (Note that where there's no fiber, as in dairy foods, there's no difference.)

FOOD	TOTAL CARBS GRAMS	AVAILABLE (NET) CARBS GRAMS
1 medium apple (5 oz)	25	18
½ cup oatmeal (porridge)	15	12
1 slice whole wheat bread	15	12
5oz (150 g) fat-free, plain Greek yogurt	7	7
1 cup (8 oz) milk*	12	12

*Fat-free, low-fat, 2 percent, and full-fat milk all contain the same carbohydrate content from the natural sugar lactose. Only the fat content changes.

CAROB SYRUP OR MOLASSES

Carob (*Ceratonia siliqua*) is a hardy, drought-resistant tree native to the eastern Mediterranean and probably the Middle East, too. It is part of the pea family. The fruit (technically a legume) has been prized since ancient times for both its gum-containing seeds and its long, dark brown pods that are rich in sugars—▶**sucrose** mostly, plus ▶**glucose**, ▶**fructose**, and ▶**maltose**.

The syrup made from the pods is a traditional topping and flavoring in Middle Eastern and Mediterranean cooking. To make it, the pods are crushed in a machine called a kibbler to separate pod pieces (kibbles) from the seeds. Nothing is wasted: the kibbles are boiled down to make syrup or processed for animal-feed products (the main use of carob pods), carob powder or flour (raw and roasted and used to make carob chips), "kibble nibbles" (a snack eaten in Australia), and carob syrup. The seeds are separately processed to make locust bean gum (also called ceratonia or carob bean gum), an additive (E410) widely used as a gelling agent, stabilizer, or emulsifier in cosmetics, pharmaceuticals, and foods.

With a flavor somewhere between ▶**molasses** and ▶**honey**, and not "chocolately" at all, the dark brown syrup is more likely to be found in an ▶**organic** or health food store or online than in a supermarket. It tends to be rather expensive, so it's best used judiciously. Drizzle it over pancakes, porridge, ice cream, yogurt, and steamed pudding; add it to hot or cold drinks (especially milky ones); try it as a mixer in creamy cocktails; use it in tangy dressings and marinades; and glaze foods with it instead of honey or ▶**maple syrup**. In baking, you may find it in ingredients list for cereal bars, cookies, moist cakes, desserts, and puddings. You may also find it combined with other syrups—we have spotted maple and carob blends.

Tip: South America's black carob syrup, made from algarobbo (*Prosopis nigra*) pods, is not the same thing. Spanish settlers called the South American tree "carob" because it reminded them of the carob tree they were so familiar with back home—and it is, in fact, from the same pea family (see also ▶**mesquite flour or powder**).

▶ CAROB SYRUP OR MOLASSES AT A GLANCE

Nutritive

Sugars Sucrose, glucose, fructose, maltose, pinitol

Sweetness relative to sucrose Less sweet (little available data)

Calories 10 calories (42 kilojoules) per level teaspoon

CASTER SUGAR

(▶superfine sugar)

Also spelled castor, this is the standard British term for superfine sugar, the finest of all ▶**granulated sugars** (▶**sucrose**), which dissolves very easily and is used in creamed cake batters and cookie doughs, meringues, and drinks. The term caster comes from the traditional silver sugar shaker that made its appearance during the latter half of the seventeenth century, by which time sugar was very much the preferred sweetener, not only added to food, but shaken over it, too. Up to this point, sugar cubes had been kept in a sugar box, but once people wanted to shake fine granules over their food, a different utensil was called for. Enter the silversmith and the silver caster. The first ones looked rather like little lighthouses—a cylinder with a detachable pierced top. Over time, they became more elaborate— embossed, engraved, and fluted. If you still have your grandmother's tea set, you may find there's a silver sugar caster sitting on the tray.

CENTRIFUGAL SUGAR

Most cane (and beet) sugars are "centrifugal sugar" products—the ▶**molasses** has been separated from the crystals in a machine you could describe essentially as a spin dryer. As the molasses-sugar crystal mixture (known, in technical terms, as *massecuite*) spins in a perforated basket, centrifugal force pushes the molasses through the holes, leaving the crystals on the basket wall. The centrifugal machine was invented by Gottfried Penzoldt, who took out a patent for it in France in 1837. His *essoreuse* (centrifuge) was designed to dry textiles.[10] Sugar refiners saw its possibilities, and it was promptly modified and widely adopted by the industry. It produced a drier sugar, which could be packed and transported in bags rather than heavier, more expensive, and cumbersome barrels that fit less neatly in the hold of a ship.

CHANCACA

This is the Peruvian name for ▶**panela**, the traditional, ▶**unrefined**, ▶**non-centrifugal sugar** still produced on family farms in small ▶**sugarcane** mills (*trapiches*) throughout Latin America and the Caribbean. It is made by slowly boiling down sugarcane juice to a thick syrup, which is either set in molds or beaten to make ▶**granulated sugar**.

CHICORY ROOT

Chicory root (*Cichorium intybus*), often used as a caffeine-free coffee substitute, is very rich in ▶**inulin**, a ▶**polysaccharide** that belongs to a class of dietary ▶**fibers** called ▶**fructans**. Inulin is found in a variety of fruits, grains, and vegetables such as bananas, wheat, onions, and garlic, but chicory root is currently the source of most of the inulin the food industry uses. As a dietary fiber, it is not digested or absorbed by the body and has no effect on ▶**blood glucose** levels, so it is found in numerous sugar-substitute products these days. However, be aware that it is not a sugar at all; it is a slightly sweet dietary fiber.

Although it shares some of ▶**granulated sugar**'s physical characteristics, such as providing bulk, it is not sufficiently sweet to replace ▶**sucrose** in recipes on a cup-for-cup basis. If you are tempted to use it in your baking, try it out first in a recipe that has been developed and tested with it (and that shows you a photograph of the end product), rather than substituting it for ▶**brown sugar** or ▶**white sugar** in one of your favorite recipes.

CHINESE ROCK SUGAR

(▶rock sugar or candy)

Rock sugar or candy, one of the oldest forms of sugar-crystal candy, originated in India and Persia. In China, its rich and subtle sweetness makes it the sugar of choice for "red cooking" (a slow-braising cooking technique), sauces, marinades, and soups such as bird's nest and dessert soups, as well as for sweetening chrysanthemum tea.

COARSE SUGAR

This specialty sugar with a large crystal size is used mainly for decoration and comes in a range of colors. *See also* ▶**decorating sugars**

COCONUT SUGAR

(coconut palm sugar, coco sap sugar, coco sugar)

This traditional, partially refined Asian sweetener is made from freshly harvested sap from the coconut palm (*Cocos nucifera*). The resulting sugar is similar in color, flavor, and sweetness to a good ▶**brown sugar**, but the texture is drier and more crumbly.

The minimal processing is much the same today as it has been for centuries. The blossom-bearing spikes (known in botanical terms as *inflorescence*) are tapped for their sweet, watery sap (around 12 percent ▶**sucrose**), which is boiled down to produce a thick syrup. This causes some of the sucrose to ▶**invert** (break down into separate ▶**glucose** and ▶**fructose** molecules). The concentrated syrup is either poured into coconut shells or bamboo molds to cool and harden into cakes or blocks, or beaten to cool and produce ▶**granulated sugar**. It takes about 2 gallons (8 liters) of sap to produce a bit over 2 pounds (1 kilogram) of coconut sugar.

Most coconut palms are multipurpose, as trees can bear up to three flowering spikes at any one time. Farmers may tap one for sap to produce sweeteners (sugar and syrup), vinegar, and beverages, including fermented alcoholic drinks (e.g., toddy and arrack), and let the remaining flowering spikes produce coconuts for other products such as coconut water, coconut milk, and coconut cream.

Although coconut sugar is sometimes promoted as a "whole food," "natural," and "healthier than regular sugar," it's still sugar and comes with the same number of calories as granulated sugar has. Thus, like all nutritive sweeteners, it may contribute to weight gain when consumed in excessive amounts, so you still have to keep your daily intake moderate. It does have a low glycemic index, but the results of the glycemic index testing carried out independently at the University of Sydney found that the glycemic index value was 54 (not the GI 35 you may find quoted frequently on the Internet).

You can use coconut sugar as a tabletop sweetener for your tea or coffee or substitute it, cup for cup, for soft brown or granulated sugar in baked goods and desserts. You can also use it when ▶**palm sugar**, ▶**jaggery**, or ▶**gur** are called for in Asian recipes. Look for it online or on the shelves of Asian produce stores and ▶**organic**, whole food, and specialty outlets. Be aware that it can vary slightly in color and flavor from batch to batch and that it is sometimes blended with ▶**cane sugar**.

▶ COCONUT SUGAR AT A GLANCE

Nutritive

Sugars Sucrose, glucose, fructose

Sweetness relative to sucrose Equally sweet

Calories 16 calories (67 kilojoules) per level teaspoon

COCONUT SYRUP OR NECTAR

To make coconut syrup, the sap from coconut palms' blossom-bearing spikes is boiled down to evaporate until the desired consistency is achieved. With its warm, toffeelike flavor, the syrup can be drizzled over cereals, oatmeal, pancakes, yogurt, ice cream, and desserts; added to hot milk drinks and cool smoothies; used to glaze sweet potatoes, squash, and meat before roasting them; and substituted on a spoon-for-spoon basis for other sweet syrups, such as ▶agave or ▶maple, in favorite recipes. *See also* ▶coconut sugar

▶ **COCONUT SYRUP OR NECTAR AT A GLANCE**
Nutritive
Sugars Sucrose, glucose, fructose
Sweetness relative to sucrose Equally sweet
Calories 14 calories (60 kilojoules) per level teaspoon (Niulife Coconut Syrup brand)

COFFEE SUGAR OR CRYSTALS

Coffee sugar is a specialty sugar crystal that is left for a longer time during the crystallizing stage of refining to form larger crystals that will dissolve more slowly in coffee and other hot drinks. They also give cookies, muffins, and other desserts an extra crunchy topping. *See also* ▶granulated sugar

▶ **COFFEE SUGAR OR CRYSTALS AT A GLANCE**
Nutritive
Sugars Sucrose
Sweetness relative to sucrose Equally sweet
Calories 16 calories (67 kilojoules) per level teaspoon (CSR Coffee Sugar Crystals brand)

CONFECTIONERS' SUGAR

(▶*powdered sugar,* ▶*icing sugar*)

This is finely ground and sifted ▶granulated sugar with a smooth texture. It dissolves readily and is used in whipped cream, icings, buttercream frostings, fondant fillings, fudge, candies, and confections;

for a final decorative dusting on cakes and desserts; and for creating glossy glazes with a smooth, satiny texture.

Although the ingredients lists in recipes will usually simply specify confectioners' (or powdered or icing) sugar, you may find an almost bewildering range of products in the supermarket. Some are the same product with an alternative name; others are slightly different products designed for specific purposes. Here is a very basic guide: Most confectioners' (powdered or icing) sugar on supermarket shelves has been blended with 3 to 4 percent cornstarch to keep it free-flowing and prevent it from clumping. It is suitable for most purposes but not for making royal icing (a smooth, hard decorator's icing). For that you need pure confectioners' (or powdered or icing) sugar with no added starch. Check the ingredients, and consider sifting pure confectioners' sugar before using it, as it does tend to get lumpy.

What about the "X factor"? You may have noticed "10-X" on packages of confectioners' sugar at the grocery store. This is the most common grade available to consumers and indicates the sugar's fineness: the more Xs, the more finely ground it is.

▶ CONFECTIONERS' SUGAR AT A GLANCE

Nutritive

Sugars Sucrose (typically also contains 4–5% cornstarch)

Sweetness relative to sucrose Equally sweet

Calories 16 calories (67 kilojoules) per level teaspoon

CORN SUGAR

Sugar produced from corn (maize) is sometimes called corn sugar and sometimes ▶**dextrose** and sometimes ▶**glucose**. In chemical terms it is glucose, a ▶**monosaccharide**. Although not as sweet, corn sugar has the same number of calories and grams of ▶**carbohydrates** per level teaspoon as ▶**granulated sugar** (▶**sucrose**) has. It also has a very high glycemic index (GI 100).

Back in 2010, producers of ▶**high fructose corn syrup (HFCS)** applied to the FDA to rename HFCS "corn sugar." They were turned down on the grounds that sugars are crystalline, and HFCS, being syrup, is liquid.

The FDA actually has a very clear definition for corn sugar as a food substance Generally Recognized As Safe (GRAS) in its *Code of*

Federal Regulations (Section 184.1857): "It occurs as the anhydrous or the monohydrate form and is produced by the complete hydrolysis of corn starch with safe and suitable acids or enzymes, followed by refinement and crystallization from the resulting hydrolysate."

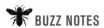 **BUZZ NOTES**

Corn Sweeteners

You may or may not have a bottle of Karo ▶**corn syrup** in your pantry, but if you live in the United States, you will probably discover that you have numerous products containing a corn sweetener on the shelf or in the fridge: it is used in salad dressings, tomato sauces, canned fruits and vegetables, powdered drink mixes, fruit drinks and juices, frozen desserts, cake mixes and frostings, and snack foods, including cookies, crackers, and pretzels. If you are label checking, look for ingredients such as "corn syrup," "▶**glucose syrup**," "corn/glucose syrup solids," "dried corn/glucose syrup," "▶**dextrose** monohydrate," "dextrous anhydrous," "▶**maltodextrin**," "high fructose corn syrup," "▶**fructose**."

Corn sweeteners are widely used by the food industry, not just because they are inexpensive, but also because they have very practical attributes—softening texture, adding volume, preventing sugar from crystallizing, and enhancing flavor. Dextrose is also used as a filler in the single-serving table-top packets of many well-known brands of artificial sweeteners.

CORN SYRUP

Here we mean regular corn syrup, not ▶**high fructose corn syrup (HFCS)**, which is a different product with different sugars and uses. Corn syrup comes from cornstarch, a powdery thickener derived from the endosperm of the corn kernel. Chemically speaking, it is a chain of glucose molecules. Corn syrup is very popular in the United States, where significantly more corn is grown than ▶**sugarcane** or ▶**sugar beet**. It's more of a rarity elsewhere in the world, which may surprise American readers.

The cornstarch-to-syrup story is very much one of American enterprise. It started back in 1806, when William Colgate opened his starch, soap, and candle business on Dutch Street in New York City. It prospered, and in 1820 he established the Wm. Colgate & Company wheat starch plant in Jersey City, New Jersey, which by 1844 evolved into the world's first dedicated cornstarch plant. Within a decade, cornstarch was big business, with its biggest customer being the laundry industry (think of all those stiff white collars and petticoats). By 1866 the factory was also using cornstarch to make ▶**glucose**, and the rest is history.

Processing cornstarch with acids or enzymes yields a syrup that is not as sweet as regular ▶**granulated sugar** but that has the same number of calories. It is used for making candy, jams, jellies, and frostings, and it is synonymous with that Southern specialty, pecan pie (so synonymous, in fact, that the pie is sometimes called *Karo nut pie*). It also adds sheen and a smooth texture to icings and caramel coatings.

In addition, corn syrup is ideal to drizzle over cereals and pancakes, use in baking, add to glazes and sauces, and sweeten beverages. In baking, it is best used in recipes that specify it as an ingredient. Substituting corn syrup for granulated sugar (▶**sucrose**) isn't simple, as you need to use more to get the same level of sweetness (which means more calories) and adjust the amount of liquid.

There are two basic varieties, based on color: light corn syrup (often with vanilla and salt added for flavor) and dark corn syrup (with added refiner's syrup, or ▶**golden syrup**, for a richer flavor). There are also reduced-calorie ("lite") versions with around one-third fewer calories per serving. Some brands also boost sweetness by adding high fructose corn syrup. *See also* ▶**glucose syrups**

▶ **CORN SYRUP AT A GLANCE**
Nutritive
Sugars Glucose, maltose
Sweetness relative to sucrose About 40% as sweet
Calories 16 calories (67 kilojoules) per level teaspoon

CURCULIN

This sweet-tasting ▶**protein** was isolated in 1990 from the tropical fruit of *Curculigo latifolia* found throughout tropical Southeast Asia, especially in Malaysia. Although the fruit itself is only slightly sweet, the protein curculin (also known as neoculin) is about 500 times sweeter than ▶**sucrose**. Although it provides 4 calories per gram, such a minute amount is required to sweeten foods that it is considered a ▶**zero-calorie (nonnutritive) sweetener**. Like ▶**miraculin**, it is a taste modifier, meaning that sour foods taste sweet after it is added. You currently won't find it listed in the ingredients list for any foods or drinks because, at the time of writing, it has not been commercialized and does not have regulatory approval for use as an additive in the United States, Australia, or Europe.

▶ **CURCULIN AT A GLANCE**
Nonnutritive
Sweetness relative to sucrose About 500 times sweeter
Calories 0
FDA approval No

CYCLAMATE

(See page 270 for brand names)

"Providence" is how chemist Dr. Michael Sveda described his chance discovery of the ▶**nonnutritive sweetener** cyclamate in 1937 while working on something completely different: a fever-reducing drug for DuPont. Introduced into foods and beverages in the 1950s, cyclamate was a billion-dollar sugar-substitute business by the 1960s for a range of reasons: the diet market was growing in the United States; food and beverage companies discovered the advantages of blending cyclamate and ▶**saccharin** to mask aftertastes; and custom cookbooks and magazines promoted the use of liquid cyclamate (Sucaryl) in cooking. Today, cyclamate is approved for use in foods and beverages in more than one hundred countries worldwide but not in the United States.

The FDA gave cyclamate GRAS status in 1958, but just over ten years later totally banned it (effective September 11, 1970) because a lab study had found that rats fed a high-dose saccharin/cyclamate mixture developed bladder tumors. Reviewing the evidence in 1984, the FDA's Cancer Assessment Committee concluded that cyclamate was not carcinogenic, and the National Academy of Sciences reaffirmed that finding in 1985.

Cyclamate has to be one of the most studied food additives. Over the past fifty years, health organizations, including the World Health Organization's Joint Expert Committee on Food Additives (JECFA) and the European Union Scientific Committee for Food (now the European Food Safety Authority, or EFSA), have regularly reviewed the evidence on cyclamate and deemed it safe for use both as a tabletop (general purpose) sweetener and as an additive in prepared foods and beverages.

Up to thirty times sweeter than regular ▶**granulated sugar**, cyclamate (technically a sodium or calcium salt of sulfamic acid) is highly soluble in liquids and heat stable in baking. Like other ▶**high-intensity sweeteners**, consumer brands of this sugar substitute come with other ingredients (usually a ▶**starch**-based sweetener, such as ▶**maltodextrin**, and cream of tartar), so check the label. It doesn't provide any calories, with up to 37 percent of ingested cyclamate being absorbed into the blood stream and passing though the body and excreted in urine without being metabolized. However, up to one in four people convert a proportion (0.1–60 percent) of the unabsorbed cyclamate into cyclohexylamine in the large intestine, which is in turn absorbed from the intestine and again excreted in the urine. Cyclohexylamine may cause bladder cancer and sexual organ pathology in animals when consumed in large amounts. Most people do not consume enough cyclamate to warrant concern.

In supermarkets around the world (but not in the United States), consumers will find cyclamate sweetening a wide range of foods and oral-hygiene products on its own or blended with (typically) saccharin. It's used in diet beverages (soft drinks, iced teas, sports drinks, and shakes); breakfast cereals; dairy products; baked goods and desserts; fruit juices, jams, jellies, and marmalades; and sauces and dressings. It is also in gum, candies, toothpaste, and mouthwash. For home use, there are packets, tablets, liquids, and white and brown granulated products you can use as a cup-for-cup sugar substitute in baking.

▶ **CYCLAMATE AT A GLANCE**
  Nonnutritive
  Sweetness relative to sucrose About 30–50 times sweeter
  Calories 0
  FDA approval No
  EFSA Number E952
  ADI 11 mg (JECFA); 7 mg (EFSA) per kilogram (2.2 pounds) of body weight
  Health Crosses placenta; may also be found in breast milk

Is it true that sugar is used in cosmetics and skin care products?

Yes, it is, especially in scrubs, rubs, soaps, exfoliators, and even bath bombs. Lush USA says that their solid, stimulating, ginger and fennel sugar scrub is "tough on cellulite and unwanted bumps, but kind on your skin. Its no-nonsense attitude doesn't waste any time getting down to business; sweetly exfoliating with ▶**Fairtrade** sugar and stimulating circulation with fennel and ginger." It's a growing market, as health-conscious consumers look for natural and animal-cruelty-free alternatives in beauty products. Along with ▶**honey**, it is possibly the oldest skin care ingredient still in use. You will find it in numerous products today, including moisturizers and face creams, packs, and masks.

DATE SYRUP OR MOLASSES

This thick, sticky, dark brown syrup (*dibis, dibs, silan*) has been enjoyed as a sweetener for thousands of years throughout the Middle
East and North Africa as an alternative to ▶**honey**; as an ingredient in
sweets, desserts, and drinks; and to balance flavors in meat and
chicken dishes. Traditionally it was made by either pressing fresh
dates to let the syrup simply ooze out (not the most productive method)
or boiling dates until they disintegrated into a pulpy mass. This mixture was then beaten, strained, and left to thicken naturally in the sun
in big containers in the summertime. In the winter, it was returned to
the pot to boil down to the desired sticky, thick consistency.

Today, many health-conscious people are looking for alternative
sweeteners that are raw or unrefined. Even though technology does
the work nowadays, date syrup is very much a minimally processed
product. The syrup is extracted from fresh and dried dates in production lines that sort, soak, stone (pit), refine, pasteurize, filter, concentrate, and bottle. The syrup is essentially "liquid dates" and is
certainly richer in vitamins—especially A and K—and minerals than
many other sweeteners, but without the ▶**fiber** of the whole date.[11]
But, despite the nutritional boost, it still comes with the same number
of calories as sugar, so it's still a don't-overdo-it food. Date syrup itself has not been glycemic index tested, although we know dried
dates have a low glycemic index (GI 39 to 45), so we would guess that
date syrup's glycemic index is low, too.

Because of its distinctive flavor (and price), date syrup is more of a
specialty than an everyday sweetener. Yotam Ottolenghi calls it the
"curveball" ingredient in the (fabulous) cookbook he wrote with Sami
Tamimi, *Jerusalem*. If you can't find it, they suggest you substitute
▶**golden syrup**, ▶**maple syrup**, or ▶**treacle** (▶**molasses**), but we don't

think these ▶**sucrose** syrups bring quite the same concentrated dried-fruit depth and richness. Date syrup comes into its own mixed with tahini as a dip, used in dressings for salads and vegetables such as roasted cauliflower or sautéed eggplant, combined with yogurt for a sweet treat or snack, or drizzled over oatmeal or pancakes. If you are not sure how to begin exploring its flavor potential, start with Ottolenghi and Tamimi's recipes (many are online). You are more likely to pick up a jar of it online or from a health food or Middle Eastern produce store than in a supermarket.

▶ DATE SYRUP OR MOLASSES AT A GLANCE

Nutritive

Sugars Glucose, fructose, sucrose

Sweetness relative to sucrose Less sweet (little available data)

Calories 16 calories (67 kilojoules) per level teaspoon

DATE SUGAR

It may look like ▶**brown sugar**, but it is not; it is powdered dried dates. Although some manufacturers suggest you can use it as a substitute for brown sugar in recipes, it's not that simple. Yes, it is sweet (dates contain contain around 70 percent sugars) but as it does not dissolve or melt, and tends to clump, it is not ideal for baking, nor for sweetening a cup of tea or coffee. It absolutely comes into its own, however, as a delicious powdery date topping to sprinkle over oatmeal or yogurt. If you do want to use it in your baking, we suggest you try it in a recipe that the manufacturer has developed with date sugar before substituting it for regular brown sugar in your favorite recipes.

Is it better for you than brown sugar? A level teaspoon of date sugar has slightly fewer calories and carbohydrates than a teaspoon of brown sugar, but it is less sweet, so you need to use more. We know dried dates have a low glycemic index (GI 39 to 45), so we would guess that date sugar's glycemic index is low, too.

As commercial varieties may have a "flowing agent" added to help prevent the powdered dates from clumping in the packet, they may not be gluten-free. Check the ingredient label. Bob's Red Mill Date Sugar, for example, also contains oat flour. As date sugar is more expensive to buy than a packet of pitted dates (and is hard to source), many people make their own. There are numerous recipes online for those who want to try.

► DATE SUGAR AT A GLANCE

Nutritive

Sugars Glucose, fructose, sucrose

Sweetness relative to sucrose Less sweet (little available data)

Calories 11 calories (46 kilojoules) per level teaspoon (Bob's Red Mill Date Sugar)

DECORATING SUGARS

Shimmers, sparkles, dusts, and sugar sheets are just part of a large and ever-evolving and ever-expanding range of sugary, candylike products that add special-occasion sparkle to cakes and cupcakes, cookies, and desserts. As you enjoy a piece of beautifully decorated birthday or wedding cake, remember that the icing or fondant and decoration are essentially concentrated sugar, and accordingly they come with a high concentration of calories, so it's probably a good idea to say "no thank you" to seconds.

DEHYDRATED CANE JUICE

"Dehydrated cane juice" and "unrefined dehydrated cane juice" are simply ways of saying sugar (►**sucrose**) in three or four words rather than one. Terms such as these fall into the marketer-confusing-the-consumer category. *See also* ►**evaporated cane juice**

DEMERARA SUGAR

Originally "demerara" was the specific name for sugar from the cane plantations on the banks of the Demerara River in today's Guyana, where it was first planted by Dutch colonists in 1746. Today, it's used as a generic term for a type of ►**raw sugar** with a dry, crunchy texture and a subtle butterscotch aroma, and it is produced by a number of cane-growing countries, but mostly Mauritius.

It is a popular tabletop sweetener in the United Kingdom, Australia, New Zealand, Canada, and, increasingly, the United States. Like ►**turbinado sugar**, its ►**molasses**-rich crystals are spun in a centrifuge to dry them, leaving coarse, light brown or tan granules. Use it to sweeten tea or coffee; sprinkle over cereals and oatmeal; add crunch to crumbles and toppings, as on crème brûlée; caramelize grilled fruit; or bring out the sweet flavor of slow-roasted tomatoes.

Chrissy Freer, who put some of the most popular alternatives to regular sugar through their baking paces in the Test Kitchen section (page 249), voted demerara her favorite for color and texture (but not looks) in both the Vanilla Butter Cookie and the Blueberry Bran Muffin recipes.

▶ **DEMERARA SUGAR AT A GLANCE**
   Nutritive
   Sugars Sucrose
   Sweetness relative to sucrose Equally sweet
   Calories 16 calories (67 kilojoules) per level teaspoon

DEXTROSE

Dextrose is another term for ▶**glucose** (D-glucose, technically), a single-sugar molecule, or ▶**monosaccharide**. The term *dextrose* is a historical one that comes from "dextrorotatory glucose" (it gets sciency here), because a solution of glucose in water rotates the plane of polarized light to the right (*dextro* means "right"). If you see dextrose in an ingredients list, it probably means that the glucose was produced from cornstarch. We explain how they convert cornstarch to sugar in our entry on glucose, but chemically, the process is not unlike the way our bodies convert starch to glucose during digestion.

DISACCHARIDE

Two single-sugar molecules joined together form a ▶**carbohydrate** called a disaccharide. *Di* means "two" and *saccharide* means "sugar." The three common dietary disaccharide sugars are:

   ▶**Lactose**, which is glucose joined with ▶**galactose**, is found in milk and yogurt. It has a low glycemic index (GI 46).
   ▶**Maltose**, which is two ▶**glucose** molecules joined together, is found in grains such as barley and in malt and malted foods and beverages. It has a high glycemic index (GI 105).
   ▶**Sucrose**, which is glucose joined with ▶**fructose**, is found in tubers such as potatoes, ▶**sugar beet**, the grass ▶**sugarcane**, the sap of ▶**maple** trees, and fruits. It has a moderate glycemic index (average GI 65).

DRIED CANE SYRUP

This is the common or usual name for the solid, or dried, form of cane syrup, according to the FDA. See ▶**evaporated cane juice** for the full story and ▶**non-centrifugal sugars** for more about these sugars and how they are made.

DULCE DE LECHE

(arequipe [Columbia, Venezuela]*, cajeta* [Mexico]*, doce de leite* [Brazil]*, manar/manjur* [Chile]*, confiture de lait* [France]*)*

Think of dulce de leche as silky, syrupy, caramelized milk rather than a sugar or sweetener per se. It is used as a filling, topping, sauce, and ingredient in desserts and baking (*alfajores*, empanadas, flans, cakes, cookies) throughout Central and South America. It's made by slowly simmering milk (e.g., cow's, goat's, or even coconut) and sugar together with a pinch of baking soda and perhaps the seeds of a vanilla bean (or a drop of pure vanilla essence) over many hours till the water in the milk has evaporated and the mixture has thickened and caramelized. Sweetened condensed milk is sometimes suggested as a substitute for dulce de leche, but the taste is not the same. These days you should be able to buy good quality, traditional dulce de leche at larger supermarkets and specialty food and produce stores, and it is available online.

Commercial dulce de leche is 70 percent solids, about a third of which are milk solids. This is why the final product provides a little protein (about 6 percent) and fat (some 7 percent) and is a source of calcium. It's not possible to estimate its glycemic index, as that would depend on the balance of sugars—dulce de leche will naturally contain ▶**sucrose** and ▶**lactose**, but manufacturers sometimes add ▶**glucose**, too.

▶ **DULCE DE LECHE AT A GLANCE**
Nutritive
Sugars Sucrose, lactose
Sweetness relative to sucrose Less sweet (varies; depends on brand or recipe used)
Calories 20 calories (84 kilojoules) per level teaspoon (Nestlé La Lechera® brand)

ERLOSE

Erlose is found naturally in ▶**honey** in small amounts. It is produced by the action of honeybee invertase (an enzyme) on ▶**sucrose**.

ERYTHRITOL

(See page 270 for brand names)

Erythritol, a ▶**polyol** (▶**sugar alcohol**) found in very small amounts in some plants (e.g., grapes, melons, and mushrooms) and fermented foods (e.g., wine, beer, sake, cheese, and soy sauce), is manufactured in commercial quantities by a fermentation process using wheat or cornstarch (maize) as a starting material. It is approved for use in foods as a ▶**bulk sweetener** in about fifty countries around the world, including the United States, the European Union, Canada, Australia, New Zealand, Brazil, and Mexico. In Japan, the earliest erythritol adopter (1990), you will find it in reduced-calorie candies, chocolate, yogurt, fillings, jellies, jams, and beverages, and it is also used as a tabletop sugar substitute.

While most polyols have a reputation for having a gassy and laxative effect, erythritol is the exception. Most (up to 90 percent) is rapidly absorbed in the small intestine and excreted unchanged in urine. Only about 10 percent enters the large intestine, where either the healthy bacteria feast on it, or it is excreted in feces. EU approval excludes beverages, as there is a concern that the laxative threshold value (see page 11) may be exceeded when it is consumed this way, especially by young people. As is the case for other polyols, the FDA has approved the claim "does not promote tooth decay" for labels on sugar-free foods containing erythritol.

Because it is only about 70 percent as sweet as ▶**granulated sugar**

(▶**sucrose**), erythritol is typically mixed with a ▶**nonnutritive sweetener** in consumer tabletop and cup-for-cup baking products, and it is these blends that have become very popular with people following low-carb, sugar-free, and paleo diets. Natvia and Zsweet, for example, are blended with ▶**stevia**, and Swerve is combined with ▶**oligosaccharides** (e.g., ▶**inulin**). As ingredients can vary depending on the application, check the label. For example, Zsweet's granulated pouches and canisters contain erythritol, stevia, and natural flavors, while their supersweet packets have all that plus calcium carbonate.

Check out manufacturers' websites for tested recipes using these blends. It is probably worthwhile to try these before experimenting and substituting an erythritol blend for sugar in one of your family favorites. Using these products will certainly help lower the overall glycemic load (impact) of your baking. But the highest glycemic index ingredient in baking is usually the flour—and, in most recipes, you can't have your cake without it.

▶ ERYTHRITOL AT A GLANCE

Nutritive

Sugars Erythritol

Sweetness relative to sucrose About 70% as sweet

Calories 0.6 calories (2.5 kilojoules) per level teaspoon (Natvia brand; varies)

FDA approval GRAS status

EFSA Number E968

ADI Not specified

LTV Not specified

Health May have laxative properties when consumed as a beverage by some people

EVAPORATED CANE JUICE

"Evaporated cane juice" is simply a way of saying "sugar" in three words rather than one, as it apparently sounds more "natural" and less like, well, sugar. You may find it listed as an ingredient on the label of some yogurts, fruit juices, and lemonades, and you may also read about it in pending lawsuits, as consumers have taken some manufacturers to court over the matter because they believe it is misleading.

Back in 2009, after "evaporated cane juice" started appearing regularly on food labels, the FDA issued a guidance suggesting that manufacturers should avoid using "evaporated cane juice" because it suggests that the sweeteners are juice, which they are not. The FDA also made the point that the common or usual name for the solid or dried form of cane syrup is "dried cane syrup." Doesn't have the same ring, does it? "Unrefined dehydrated cane juice" is another term that we think comes into the marketer-confusing-the-consumer category. It, too, is partially refined ▶**sucrose**.

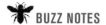 **BUZZ NOTES**

What the FDA Says About Evaporated Cane Juice

The FDA's 2009 draft guidance (nonbinding recommendations) suggest that:

"Sweeteners derived from sugarcane syrup should not be listed in the ingredient declaration by names which suggest that the ingredients are juice, such as 'evaporated cane juice.' FDA considers such representations to be false and misleading under section 403(a) (1) of the Act (21 U.S.C. 343(a)(1)) because they fail to reveal the basic nature of the food and its characterizing properties (i.e., that the ingredients are sugars or syrups) as required by 21 CFR 102.5. Furthermore, sweeteners derived from sugarcane syrup are not juice and should not be included in the percentage juice declaration on the labels of beverages that are represented to contain fruit or vegetable juice (see 21 CFR 101.30)."[12]

FAIRTRADE SUGAR AND SWEETENERS

The international Fairtrade certification mark on a package of sugar and other sweeteners is a guarantee that the frequently disadvantaged farmers and workers in the developing world who produced it received a fair price for it and are getting a better deal overall. For example, sugar farmers who sell to the Fairtrade market are members of local agricultural co-ops, which receive a premium to help fund community development programs such as improving the water supply, providing schooling and health care, and purchasing harvesting equipment. For more information, see fairtrade.net/sugar.html.

FIBER

Dietary fibers are large ►**carbohydrate** molecules made up of many different sorts of ►**monosaccharides**. Unlike ►**starches** and sugars, they are not broken down during digestion by humans. They come mostly (but not exclusively) from plants and are the poorly digested portions that pass through into the large intestine (bowel) and provide much of the bulk in our stools (along with water and bacteria, among other things).

FODMAPS

FODMAPs—**F**ermentable **O**ligosaccharides, **D**isaccharides, **M**onosaccharides, **A**nd **P**olyols—are sugars that can be poorly absorbed in some people's intestines and cause symptoms such as abdominal pain and discomfort, bloating, gas, distention, and altered bowel habits. These sugars are found in a wide range of foods and drinks, such as:

> ►**Fructans**
> ►**Fructooligosaccharides**—found in wheat, rye, onions, and garlic

Galactooligosaccharides—found in legumes

▶**Fructose**—found in fruit and ▶**honey**

▶**Lactose**—found in milk and milk products

▶**Polyols**—such as ▶**sorbitol** and ▶**mannitol**, found in some fruits and vegetables and in processed foods where they are used as sugar-replacers and bulking agents

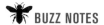 **BUZZ NOTES**

The Low-FODMAP Diet

The low-▶**FODMAP** diet is a diet developed to help people suffering from common digestive illnesses such as irritable bowel syndrome (IBS). The researchers report that 75 percent of people with IBS have greatly improved symptoms when they remove FODMAP-rich foods from their diet.[13]

FONDANT ICING SUGAR

Some manufacturers produce a ▶**confectioners' sugar** specifically for making fondant and edible cake decorations. Like ▶**powdered sugar**, it may contain cornstarch to prevent caking and increase shelf life.

FRUCTANS

Fructans are a type of soluble dietary ▶**fiber** (which means zero calories). In simple terms, a fructan is a chain of ▶**fructose** molecules joined together. The category is divided into ▶**fructooligosaccharides** and galactooligosaccharides. All fructans count as ▶**FODMAPs** and may, therefore, cause digestive distress for certain people.

FRUCTOMALTOSE

Fructomaltose has recently been found to occur naturally in ▶**honeydew**, the rich, sticky liquid secreted by aphids and some scale insects as they feed on plant sap.

FRUCTOOLIGOSACCHARIDES AND FRUCTANS

(▶oligofructose)

Fructooligosaccharides are not actually sweeteners; they are fructans found in ▶agave, artichokes, asparagus, bananas, carrots, ▶**chicory root**, garlic, Jerusalem artichokes, jicama, leeks, onions, wheat, and ▶**yacon**.

Short-chain fructans (fructooligosaccharides) are about 30 percent as sweet as ▶**granulated sugar** (▶**sucrose**). Longer-chain fructans (▶**inulin**) are about 10 percent as sweet as granulated sugar.

Fructooligosaccharides are used to replace part of the sugar (sucrose, ▶**glucose**, or ▶**fructose**) in reduced-calorie foods and beverages. Chicory root and Jerusalem artichoke are the main sources of fructooligosaccharides used in the food industry. They have a prebiotic effect, which means they are good for digestive health. However, they may not be suitable for people who are following a low-▶**FODMAP** diet due to digestive problems such as irritable bowel syndrome (IBS).

FRUCTOSE

(fruit sugar)

Abundant in nature as the main sugar in fruits, berries, ▶**honey**, flowers, most root vegetables, and some grains, fructose has provided energy for humans, birds, and mammals for millions of years. These days, it is superabundant in the supermarket, as well. When you put regular soft drinks and sweetened foods such as yogurt, dairy-based and frozen desserts, breads, cookies, cake mixes, salad dressings, mayonnaise, sauces (e.g., tomato), and some soups (again, e.g., tomato) into your shopping cart, chances are you will be adding fructose to your diet in the form of ▶**sucrose** (50 percent fructose and 50 percent ▶**glucose** from ▶**sugarcane** or ▶**sugar beet**) or ▶**high fructose corn syrup** (typically 55 percent fructose and 45 percent glucose). Regular ▶**corn syrup** does not contain fructose.

Discovered in 1847 by French chemist Augustin-Pierre Dubrunfaut, fructose is a ▶**monosaccharide** that is used as a ▶**nutritive sweetener**. It has slightly fewer calories than ▶**granulated sugar** (sucrose) and is about 70 percent sweeter, so you can use less and therefore cut back your calorie intake when you use it as a substitute. It also has a very low glycemic index (GI 19) because it is absorbed from the small intestine and taken directly to the liver, where it is immediately metabolized, and only a small proportion (20 percent) is converted to glucose and released back into the bloodstream. By comparison, most sucrose-based sugars have a glycemic index of 65 (on average). Most of the fructose is converted by the liver into the starch glycogen (see page 77), for storage, or into pyruvate and released into the blood. In humans, less than 1 percent of a given dose of fructose is converted directly into triglycerides. (Fat travels in our bloodstream as a triglyceride.)

Fructose malabsorption can be a problem for some people. It occurs when fructose is consumed without glucose, because the small intestine is impaired in its ability to absorb fructose alone, although scientists do not yet understand why this is so. If fructose is not absorbed properly in the small intestine, it can travel through to the large intestine, where bacteria ferment it, sometimes causing bloating, gas, pain, nausea, diarrhea, and/or constipation. Most people experience fructose malabsorption if they consume more than 50 grams (10 teaspoons) in one dose.

Pure crystalline fructose, typically derived from corn, is available as a tabletop sweetener. It tastes like ▶**regular sugar**, but you use around one-third less. If you want to substitute it for sugar in your baking, our advice would be to check out the recipes on the manufacturers' websites first; you may also need to lower the oven temperature slightly or reduce the baking time, since browning is more rapid. Now Foods (nowfoods.com) suggests that "you will need to experiment a little in order to determine the exact amount of fructose needed to substitute for table sugar in a recipe. In general, if a recipe calls for 1 cup of sugar, a little over ⅔ cup of fructose should be equivalent, but sweetening to taste will yield the best results. . . . Since a smaller volume of fructose than sugar would be needed in a recipe, you may have to increase the dry ingredients proportionally to compensate."

▶ FRUCTOSE AT A GLANCE

Nutritive

Sugars Fructose

Sweetness relative to sucrose About 70% sweeter

Calories 10 calories (42 kilojoules) per level teaspoon

Health Contains ▶FODMAPs

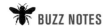 **BUZZ NOTES**

Fructose and Weight Gain

Concerned people who believe there is a simple, magic-bullet solution to obesity and weight gain have zealously blamed sugars in general and ▶**fructose** in particular. An independent assessment of all the scientific evidence regarding fructose and weight gain published in the prestigious journal *Annals of Internal Medicine* found that:

- Fructose (whether naturally occurring, as in fruit, or added, as in a soft drink) is no more likely to cause weight gain than any other form of sugars or ▶**starches** in diets that provide the same number of calories.
- There is a modest amount of weight gain (about 0.5 kg/1 pound) when large amounts of pure fructose (25 teaspoons or more) are consumed in addition to all the foods and drinks a person would normally eat.
- When eaten in the form of fruit, fructose helps people lose weight.[14]

"The reality is that the state of our health is not about any one thing," says Dr. David Katz, president of the American College of Lifestyle Medicine. "We can cut fat and get fatter and sicker—by eating more starchy, sugary junk. We can cut carbs by switching from beans to baloney and get fatter and sicker. And we can cut sugar and consume ever more artificially sweetened, starchy, fatty junk—and get fatter and sicker. We clearly like little bits of truth we find easy to digest. But none of these is the whole truth, and when bits of truth are mistaken for the whole—they might just as well be falsehoods."[15]

FRUIT CONCENTRATES

Concentrated forms of fruit juice are made by evaporating most of the water and thus concentrating the natural sugars, which will be some combination of ▶**fructose**, ▶**glucose**, and ▶**sucrose**, depending on the fruit. Some brands add back the pulp for extra ▶**fiber**, and some add back the aroma. You can use them in place of other liquid sweeteners or ▶**honey** in your cooking and baking or drizzle them over breakfast cereal, oatmeal, plain yogurt, or pancakes as a sweetener that brings a few vitamins (as well as calories) to the table.

Is it okay to drink fruit juices, or are they just more added sugars?

Drinking half a glass (4 fluid ounces/125 milliliters/½ cup) of pure fruit juice (with no added sugars) can be an effective way to boost your (or your child's) fruit intake. It counts as one serving of fruit. (A serving of fruit is about the amount that fits in the palm of your hand.)

The problem with juice, however, is that it's all too easy to overdo it, because fruit juice is rich in natural sugars and calories. For example, a "jumbo" orange juice may contain the equivalent of ten oranges, which is five times the two servings a day recommended in dietary guidelines.

You also miss out on one of the big benefits of whole fruit—the skin (or the fibrous material next to it), which is normally discarded during juicing. This contains much of the fruit's ▶**fiber** and trace minerals, along with some of its protective antioxidants.

While we would not go as far as to say that the natural sugars in juice are "added sugars," we do suggest you keep your intake moderate—one serving a day is appropriate for most of us.

And don't make it the only way you get two fruits and five veggies into you. One clear benefit from consuming fruit and vegetables the traditional way (i.e., eating them) is that it takes longer than drinking. Chewing food takes time, and taking time over food helps you manage your appetite, feel fuller longer, and avoid overeating.

Does the high amount of fructose in juice have any negative effects?

As Jennie Brand-Miller explains, when it comes to any sugary product (natural or otherwise), you have a mixture of sugars including ▶**sucrose**, ▶**glucose**, and ▶**fructose** in fruits and fruit juices. On average, the ratio of fructose to glucose is about 1:1 in most foods, including fruits and fruit juices. Sucrose is digested quickly to glucose plus fructose before absorption. The fructose is metabolized in the liver, and most is converted to glucose and burned as a source of fuel or stored as glycogen (see page 77). While glucose is generally absorbed rapidly, absorption can be slowed by acidic solutions (e.g., fruits, which are all acidic) and very concentrated solutions. If fructose is consumed on its own, the process of absorption is slower, and some may escape absorption. The presence of glucose increases the rate of absorption of fructose. The fructose in fruit and fruit juice is one reason they have a low GI. But it's not the only reason. The old adage applies: enjoy in moderation.[16]

FRUIT MOLASSES OR SYRUP

Making a fruit molasses or syrup by boiling and concentrating fruit juice goes way back to ancient times. Before sugar became available or affordable, fruit molasses provided an alternative source of sweetness to ▶honey, especially throughout the winter months. In grape-growing areas, the molasses or syrup might typically be made from grapes, and in date-growing areas from dates. But other fruits were used, as well, such as figs, mulberries, plums, apples, pears, ▶sugar beets, watermelon, and pomegranates. *See also* ▶carob syrup; ▶date syrup; ▶grape syrup; ▶pomegranate molasses

GALACTOSE

This is a ▶**monosaccharide** mostly found in milk, yogurt, and whey that is 40 percent less sweet than ▶**sucrose**. When combined with ▶**glucose**, it forms the ▶**disaccharide** ▶**lactose**, or milk sugar. Some people have a rare inherited disorder called galactosemia, which means that they are unable to fully break down galactose. It affects about 1 in 60,000 Caucasian babies and generally becomes apparent in the first few weeks of life, because they are unable to digest breast milk (lactose) or regular infant formulas. However, they are able to digest ▶**fructose**-based formulas. To find out more about it, check out the Galactosemia Foundation's website: galactosemia.org.

▶ **GALACTOSE AT A GLANCE**
Nutritive
Sugars Galactose
Sweetness relative to sucrose About 60% as sweet
Calories 16 calories (67 kilojoules) per level teaspoon

GLUCITOL

See ▶sorbitol

GLUCOSE AND GLUCOSE SYRUPS

(▶*dextrose*)

Glucose is a ▶**monosaccharide** naturally found in some fruits, some vegetables, and the nectar and sap of plants. It is also part of the ▶**disaccharides** ▶**maltose** (two glucose molecules), ▶**sucrose** (glucose plus ▶**fructose**), and ▶**lactose** (glucose plus ▶**galactose**); and three to nine glucose molecules linked in chains make up ▶**maltodextrins**—▶**oligosaccharides** used as food additives.

Our bodies need energy to work, and glucose provides it. It is a major source of energy for our cells and the primary fuel for our energy-hungry brain and for a growing fetus (see Buzz Notes, page 76). The body stores leftover glucose in the liver and muscles as glycogen, a backup energy source (see page 77). Excess glucose can also be converted to and stored as fat, which can later be broken down and used as an energy source (this is the basis for the virtually carb-free, ketogenic first phase of numerous diets).

The origins of the glucose industry go back over two hundred years to Russia, when German chemist Konstantin Kirchoff showed three flasks to the Russian Imperial Academy of Science in Saint Petersburg. Glucose industry expert Peter Hull tells us that "one flask contained syrup produced artificially from vegetables (potatoes, wheat, and buckwheat). The second contained some 'sugar' obtained from this very syrup by drying, and the third contained a syrup made from the 'dried sugar'. . . . the different vegetables had been heated with sulphuric acid to obtain the syrup."[17]

In 1814, Nicolas-Théodore de Saussure showed that the syrups produced by Kirchoff contained glucose.

No one seems to know exactly why Kirchoff carried out these experiments or what he was trying to achieve. But because of the Napoleonic Wars, Kirchoff's work was adopted "on a large scale in the Russian Empire, as the price of cane sugar had increased so much and the supply was so uncertain."[18]

Although not as sweet as ▶**granulated sugar** (sucrose), glucose has essentially the same number of calories and grams of ▶**carbohydrates** per level teaspoon. It also has a high glycemic index (GI 100), and it was, therefore, chosen for use as the reference food in glycemic index testing following the international standard method. As an ingredient, it is probably more widely used by the food industry (in sweets, ice creams, fruit preparations, brewing, baking, ketchups, sauces, and cough syrups) than by consumers in general home cooking or as a tabletop sweetener. People who need (or wish) to avoid fructose may keep a packet of glucose (dextrose) in their fructose-free pantry, and home brewers sometimes use it as a ▶**priming sugar**.

Apart from glucose (usually corn) syrups, you can purchase 100 percent pure glucose in tablets and powder form in products such as Glucodin—promoted as a quick-digesting energy top-up for very active people, as well as for listless convalescents with no appetite who need calories and an energy boost. The tablets are also used by people with type 1 diabetes who feel "a hypo" coming on (meaning, hypoglycemia, when the ▶**blood glucose** level/BGL has dropped too low) and need to eat or drink food with a high level of glucose immediately to prevent their BGL from dropping further.

Glucose is typically the sugar included in oral rehydration solutions, which are drinks specially designed for babies and young children who become dehydrated through vomiting and/or diarrhea. These special drinks help replenish fluids and electrolytes that have been lost, as well as provide an energy source (that's where the glucose comes in) until the baby or toddler can return to a normal diet. Worldwide, diarrheal diseases are a leading cause of mortality in children under five. Because the immediate cause of death in most cases is dehydration, these deaths are almost entirely preventable if dehydration is prevented or treated.

▶ GLUCOSE AND GLUCOSE SYRUPS AT A GLANCE
Nutritive
Sugars Glucose
Sweetness relative to sucrose About 70% as sweet
Calories 16 calories (67 kilojoules) per level teaspoon

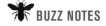 BUZZ NOTES
We Are Powered by Glucose

Like plants, we rev on ▶**glucose**. It fuels all our body cells, our brains, and our red blood cells and gives our muscles the energy they need during strenuous exercise. It comes from the carbs we eat that are broken down into glucose during digestion. It also fuels a growing fetus. Here's what Dr. Jennie Brand-Miller says in her book *The Low GI Eating Plan for an Optimal Pregnancy*:

> Pregnancy is a stage in life when the carbohydrates in food play a starring role. This is because your average blood glucose level throughout the day is directly correlated with your baby's growth rate in the womb. Quite simply, glucose is the primary fuel that drives all aspects of your baby's development. If your glucose levels are too high, then your baby will grow too fast and be born with excessive amounts of body fat. This is not a new finding. It's the

main reason why women who have type 1 diabetes (a condition that requires daily insulin injections to maintain normal glucose levels) are given close medical attention before and during their pregnancies. It's also the principal reason why all pregnant women are routinely screened during pregnancy to determine if they have developed gestational diabetes. What's new is that we now know that even mildly elevated glucose levels during pregnancy can have serious consequences.

Even if you are healthy and well, if your glucose levels are too low, your baby's growth might be too slow for its own good. Conversely, if your blood glucose levels tend to be on the high side, your baby will grow rapidly and become too big for its own good (not to mention yours!). An overly large baby is linked to greater risk of delivery complications for both mother and baby. These infants have an increased risk of childhood obesity, as well as a higher risk of metabolic diseases such as type 2 diabetes and hypertension in adulthood. As usual, moderation is a good thing.[19]

What's glycogen?

Our bodies can store a certain amount of excess ▶**carbohydrates** (about 1,500 to 1,900 calories worth) in the liver and muscles as a kind of ▶**starch** known as glycogen. One way to think of glycogen is as an energy reservoir we can draw on when going without food for a long time or exercising intensely. That's when our bodies convert it back to glucose to provide energy for our bodies and brains. Athletes restore glycogen by consuming carbohydrates on a regular basis because their supply becomes depleted as the intensity and duration of their exercise increases. In high-intensity sports, it is generally the availability of carbohydrate stores that limits performance.

Low ▶**blood glucose** occurs during exercise when the muscle uptake of ▶**glucose** is greater than the production of glucose. The effect of exercise can last as long as 72 hours after the exercise is over unless the exercise is a form of high-intensity exercise such as spinning. High-intensity exercise causes a hormone reaction that releases glucose quickly.

GLYCYRRHIZIN

(glycyrrhizic acid; glycyrrhizinic acid)

Glycyrrhizin is about fifty to one hundred times sweeter than ▶**sucrose** with a refreshing, licoricelike aftertaste, which is not surprising, as it is extracted from the long, thick root (up to 40 inches/ 1 meter long) of *Glycyrrhiza glabra* ("sweet root"), better known as licorice. It is not approved as a sugar substitute in the United States, but it is Generally Recognized As Safe (GRAS) as a flavoring or flavor enhancer in foods, beverages, sweets, and pharmaceuticals.

The European Union's Scientific Committee on Food recommends licorice lovers stick to an upper daily intake of 100 milligrams for all licorice products—equivalent to eating a couple of ounces of black licorice a day. This is because glycyrrhizin has a downside: when consumed in large quantities, it can cause potassium levels in the body to fall and blood pressure to rise. Many "licorice" or "licorice flavor" products, however, do not contain any licorice. Instead, they contain anise oil, which has the same smell and taste. In addition, deglycyrrhizinated licorice (DGL) has been manufactured to avoid the side effects of licorice by removing the active compound glycyrrhizin.

▶ GLYCYRRHIZIN AT A GLANCE

Nonnutritive

Sweetness relative to sucrose About 50–100 times sweeter

Calories 0

FDA approval GRAS status (as a flavoring)

EFSA Number E958

Health Can reduce blood potassium levels when consumed in large doses (greater than 100 mg), leading to edema

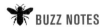 BUZZ NOTES

Licorice Can Also Help Digestive Complaints—Now, That's Sweet.

According to Natural Medicines Comprehensive Database, a database that rates the effectiveness of products and drugs based on evidence, licorice is possibly effective for significantly reducing reflux (also called heartburn). It is also used for digestive complaints including stomach ulcers, colic, and ongoing inflammation of the lining of the stomach. There are compounds in licorice that are believed to increase local prostaglandin levels, promoting mucus secretion and cell production in the stomach. Natural Medicines Comprehensive Database says 3 grams per day of licorice for up to 3 to 4 weeks is likely safe when taken by healthy adults. Make sure you get the DGL form of licorice; DGL stands for deglycyrrhizinated, and it means it is licorice without glycyrrhizin, the ingredient that might raise blood pressure.

What about safety?

■ It's always important to first talk to your health care provider if you plan to start using licorice to treat a medical problem, as it might interfere with prescription medicines.

■ If you take steroids or have high blood pressure, heart disease, hormone-sensitive conditions such as breast cancer, or kidney disease, DO NOT take licorice, because it might affect potassium or hormone levels in your body or change how the liver breaks down some medications.

But if you are a healthy adult, 700 to 800 mg chewable tablets of DGL licorice might be just what your stomach needs. For more information, visit nlm.nih.gov/medlineplus/druginfo/natural/881.html.

GOLDEN, GOLDEN BROWN, AND GOLDEN YELLOW SUGARS

A great deal of "mingling" (their word) goes on in sugar refineries to produce what manufacturers call "specialty" sugars for the marketplace—essentially anything other than regular refined white ▶**granulated sugar** or ▶**raw sugar**. We aren't going to stick our necks out and say whether these light ▶**brown sugars** are ▶**white sugar** (▶**sucrose**) sprayed with a thin coating of ▶**molasses** syrup or brown all through (i.e., with the molasses left in during refining). It depends on the brand and the type. What we can say is that, one way or another, they have enough molasses to give them a subtle caramel color and flavor. The "golden" range includes regular granulated sugar, ▶**superfine sugar,** and ▶**confectioners' sugar.**

GOLDEN SYRUP

For some of our readers, golden syrup will be dripping with childhood memories. If you grew up in Australia or New Zealand, you will remember hanging around the kitchen when Anzac biscuits were being baked just so you could lick the sticky spoon used to add the golden syrup to the mixing bowl.

Thick, velvety golden syrup was no chance discovery. It was the brainchild of Scottish businessman Abram Lyle, who encouraged Charles Eastick, his chemist, to develop the treacly by-product of sugar refining into something he could sell, rather than waste. The first customers for "Goldie," the resulting new syrup, were Lyle's employees and locals. But word spread fast. By 1885, Lyle's green and gold tins were to be found in grocery stores all over Britain, and golden syrup soon became big business for Lyle's. The syrup proved handy for provisioning troops and explorers—ancient tins of Lyle's Golden Syrup sit frozen in time inside Captain Robert Falcon Scott's base camp hut in Antarctica.

Golden syrup (sometimes called refiner's syrup) is "partially inverted sugar syrup" made from blended ▶**sugarcane** syrups (▶**sucrose** and ▶**invert sugar**). We discuss invert sugar in more detail elsewhere, but it is essentially sucrose (a ▶**disaccharide**) that has been split (inverted) into its component ▶**glucose** and ▶**fructose** ▶**monosaccharide** molecules. The advantage of the blend is that it crystallizes less readily than a pure sucrose solution.

There are numerous brands of golden syrup, but if you want the real thing, check that the label says "pure cane sugar," as some blends use ▶**corn syrup**. It is typically used at the table to drizzle over porridge, pancakes, and flapjacks. As an ingredient, it stars in such traditional British-style desserts as steamed suet and sticky puddings; ▶**treacle** tart and treacle sponge pudding; oaty cookies such as Anzac biscuits; and sweets such as hokey pokey (a Cornish term for honeycomb), in which it reduces the risk of the boiling sugar mixture crystallizing. A good quality, runny ▶**honey** is probably the best substitute for golden syrup in recipes.

▶ GOLDEN SYRUP AT A GLANCE

Nutritive

Sugars Glucose, fructose, sucrose

Sweetness relative to sucrose About 25% sweeter

Calories 16 calories (67 kilojoules) per level teaspoon

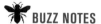

BUZZ NOTES
Anzac Biscuits

Anzac biscuits are a beloved tradition for Australians and New Zealanders, who make these eggless cookies from oats and ▶**golden syrup** every year to commemorate Anzac Day, April 25. *ANZAC* stands for "Australian and New Zealand Army Corps"–originally meaning the soldiers from Australia and New Zealand who landed at Gallipoli in April 1915; later it came to refer to any Australian or New Zealand World War I soldier. How the cookies got to be called Anzac is unclear and highly contested (and we are speaking potential international conflict here). However, cookbooks from the 1920s in both Australia and New Zealand typically had a recipe for them (with or without coconut). Here's a 1926 recipe (without coconut):

Ingredients: 2 cups rolled oats, ½ cup sugar, 1 cup plain flour, ½ cup melted butter, 1 tablespoon golden syrup, 2 tablespoons boiling water, 1 teaspoon baking soda (add a little more water if mixture is too dry)

Method: Combine dry ingredients. Mix golden syrup, boiling water, and baking soda until they froth. Add melted butter. Combine butter mixture and dry ingredients. Drop teaspoons of mixture on floured tray, allowing room for spreading. Bake in a slow oven [300–325°F/150–160°C].[20]

GRANULATED SUGAR

(▶regular sugar, ▶table sugar, ▶white sugar)

Once a luxury commodity described as "white gold," granulated sugar, with its clean, sweet taste, is today's all-purpose pantry staple for sugar and mixing bowls. It is the most common household form of sugar, with fine crystals that are easy to measure out, cream into batters, sprinkle over foods, and dissolve in drinks. Although mostly thought of as simply a sweetener, regular table sugar is much more. It is a versatile workhorse that acts as a preservative in many foods, gels with pectin in jams and jellies, and adds volume, texture, and color to baked goods and desserts.

Regular white table sugar, which is refined from ▶**sugarcane** or ▶**sugar beet**, is ▶**sucrose**—the yardstick by which all other sweeteners are measured. Sugars that are less sweet than sucrose are: ▶**lactose** (about 40 percent as sweet), ▶**maltose** (about 30 to 50 percent as sweet), and ▶**glucose** (about 70 percent as sweet); ▶**fructose**, on the other hand, is about 70 percent sweeter. The ▶**nonnutritive sweeteners** that you can buy for tabletop and household use are significantly sweeter than sucrose, ranging from ▶**aspartame** (150 to 250 times sweeter) to ▶**stevia** (200 times sweeter), ▶**saccharin** (300 to 500 times sweeter), and ▶**sucralose** (400 to 600 times sweeter).

Sucrose is a ▶**disaccharide** composed of 50 percent fructose and 50 percent glucose molecules. Nutritionally, it provides calories and carbohydrates but little else. Like other ▶**carbohydrates**, it will contribute to cavities if you don't brush your teeth regularly with a fluoride toothpaste, and weight gain if you eat too much of it. As for diabetes, there's international consensus among medical health researchers and scientists specializing in diabetes that sugar does not cause it. (See page 227 for more details.) Granulated sugar typically has a moderate glycemic index (GI 65).

▶ **GRANULATED SUGAR AT A GLANCE**

Nutritive

Sugars Sucrose

Calories 16 calories (67 kilojoules) per level teaspoon

GRAPE SYRUP OR MOLASSES

Unfermented grape juice, slowly reduced over many hours, yields a concentrated, syrupy sweetener that has been used since classical times and an aromatic, velvety condiment that complements both sweet and savory dishes. If you head for the store to buy some, you have a number of options. You may find grape syrup or molasses (▶**pekmez** or *petimezi*) in Middle Eastern, Turkish, Greek, kosher/Israeli, or specialty food stores or online. But you can also head to a well-stocked, high-end supermarket and put a bottle of probably pricey but more readily available ▶**vincotto** (**vino cotto**) or ▶**saba** into your shopping basket (we found it near the balsamic vinegars, not the syrups). Make sure it's the real thing. The only ingredient should be "grape must" and, if flavored, whatever fruit it has been infused with—typically figs, apples, or quince.

For the Romans, boiling down unfermented grape juice, or "must," was another way to make the most of the annual grape harvest. Their syrups came in various consistencies (*defrutum*, *carenum*, and *sapa*), and they added them to wine (to improve the flavor) and to meat and fruit dishes. It is reported that the syrups were also fed to pigs and ducks to make them tastier to eat.

From dressing salads to drizzling over roasted vegetables, glazing meats, or topping ice cream, these syrups make a versatile addition to a wide variety of dishes. Using the syrup to deglaze pans adds an irresistible sweetness to the resulting sauce. For day-to-day use, when you want to keep things quick and easy, simply combine it with tahini as a dip or use instead of other tabletop syrups, such as ▶**maple syrup**, with yogurt, oatmeal, pancakes, or waffles.

▶ GRAPE SYRUP OR MOLASSES AT A GLANCE

Nutritive

Sugars Glucose and fructose (proportions vary depending on ripeness and grape variety)

Sweetness relative to sucrose About 10% sweeter (Chateau Barossa brand grape syrup)

Calories 16 calories (67 kilojoules) per level teaspoon

GUR

Gur, another name for ▶**jaggery,** is the "first-stage," partially refined, ▶**non-centrifugal sugar** made from ▶**sugarcane** and the sap of various ▶**palm** trees in south and southeast Asia.

What's the difference between gur and jaggery?

They are one and the same—the unrefined, ▶**non-centrifugal sugar** produced from ▶**sugarcane** or from ▶**palm** trees. *Gur* is from the Sanskrit *guḍa* (or *gula*) for "to make into a ball." *Jaggery,* which is probably the better-known term internationally, is from the Portuguese *xagara,* from the Sanskrit *śarkarā,* meaning "sugar." J. H. Galloway, in *The Sugar Cane Industry: An Historical Geography from Its Origins to 1914,* tells us that dating the beginning of the manufacture of sugar in northern India hinges on the etymology of these two Sanskrit words. Sadly, we can't be more precise than somewhere "between the seventh and fourth centuries BC," although we know from Sanskrit hymns from the Vedic period that sugarcane was being cultivated in northern India possibly as early as 1500 BC.[21]

HIGH FRUCTOSE CORN SYRUP (HCFS)

▶**Corn syrup** is often found in the ingredients list of American processed foods and beverages. It is the most common form of sweetener in North America because it is cheaper than ▶**cane sugar**—corn farmers in the United States receive huge federal subsidies, whereas sugar importers pay tariffs. Corn syrup is made from cornstarch by enzymatic or chemical treatment. Further treatment produces high fructose corn syrup.

High fructose corn syrup is actually a misnomer, because this sweetener typically doesn't contain high fructose levels. The name comes from the fact that pure corn syrup contains no fructose at all, but treatment with enzymes obtains varying proportions of fructose. These are the most common HFCS products:

HFCS-55 (55 percent ▶**fructose** and 45 percent ▶**glucose**, on average) is mostly used in beverages such as soft drinks.

HFCS-42 (42 percent fructose and 58 percent glucose, on average) is used in many solid foods and baked goods.

HFCS-90 (90 percent fructose) and crystalline fructose (99.5 percent fructose or higher) are also produced for specialty applications.

Consumption of HFCS has risen significantly in the United States since the 1970s, when sugar tariffs and quotas increased the cost of imported sugar, and food and beverage manufacturers looked for cheaper sources of equivalent sweetness. This increase has run parallel to the increase in obesity in the country up until 2000. However, while fructose may be one factor associated with this particular obesity epidemic (think of all those extra calories, for starters), it is unlikely that it is a major factor in the obesity epidemics elsewhere. For example, Australians are getting fatter, too, but HFCS is not used at all in food and beverage production there, and total and added fructose intakes have actually decreased in Australia.[22]

What about its glycemic index? To date, no HFCS manufacturer has published its GI test data, but we know the GI of fructose and glucose, so we estimate that HFCS-55 has GI 56 and that HFCS-42 has GI 66.

▶ HIGH FRUCTOSE CORN SYRUP AT A GLANCE

Nutritive

Sugars Fructose, glucose

Sweetness relative to sucrose HFCS-55 about 160% sweeter; HFCS-42 about 120% sweeter

Calories 16 calories (67 kilojoules) per level teaspoon

HIGH-INTENSITY SWEETENERS (HIS)

(▶artificial sweeteners; ▶nonnutritive sweeteners; ▶zero-calorie sweeteners; see page 270 for brand names)

High-intensity sweeteners are food additives that are much, much sweeter than ▶**sucrose**, which means they can be used in minute amounts. They are added to foods to provide sweetness without calories (or with minimal calories). Most products labeled "diet," "diabetic-friendly," or "zero calories"—including soft drinks, yogurts, pudding, Jell-O, breath mints, and gum—contain high-intensity sweeteners.

HONEY

Ancient rock art in Spain depicts our forebears braving wild bees to steal honeycomb; Éric Valli's extraordinary *National Geographic* images display Nepali men harnessed by ropes to cliff-hugging ladders to rob the Himalayan cliff bees of their honey; Indigenous Australian women used to capture a bee, attach a feather to its body so they could track it back to the hive, remove the hive's contents (honey, wax, and bees), and eat everything; and a David Attenborough YouTube video shows a Hadza man in Tanzania following the honeyguide bird to a hive hidden in the rocks and smoking out the stinging bees to get the honey. All these instances suggest that honey has long been very desirable to humankind (and we would go to great lengths to get it).

Certainly, the nutritional benefits are clear: Honey provides a quick source of calories and ▶**carbohydrates**, and it is easy to transport and store. Wild honey also has traces of bee larvae, which add fat, protein, vitamins, and minerals. Today, we know that honey also contains antioxidants.

Despite having a sweet ending, there's no doubt that early encounters with hives full of stinging bees were likely to have been rather painful until our ancestors learned how to control fire and smoke the bees to calm (and divert or preoccupy) them. At some point, people realized there had to be an easier way to ensure a regular supply of honey. Thus began apiculture—the art of beekeeping. We don't know exactly when, but a carving from an Egyptian temple dating back around 4,500 years shows men collecting honeycombs from cylindrical containers, pouring honey into jars, and possibly separating honey from beeswax. In the ruins of Tel Rehov in Israel's Beth-Shean Valley, archaeologists have excavated thirty straw and unbaked-clay hives dating back 3,000 years. They estimate the apiary would have contained around a hundred hives for a town with a population of about two thousand residents.

If you like to sweeten your food or drinks with honey or use it in your cooking, you are following a very long tradition. The sweetness you enjoy comes from ▶**fructose** and ▶**glucose**. Most honeys have more fructose than glucose—typically 38 percent fructose to 30 percent glucose—but that's not set in stone. It all depends on where the bees have been buzzing, which is also why honey's sweetness can vary: some are equal in sweetness to regular ▶**granulated sugar** (▶**sucrose**); others are up to 50 percent sweeter. To achieve consistent sweetness and flavor (and price), most commercial honeys are made from a mixture of honeys derived from different hives and different floral sources.

We are often asked by readers of our monthly free online newsletter, *GI News*, whether honey is a better sweetener choice than regular sugar when it comes to ▶**blood glucose** levels. Again, it depends very much on what blossom the bees were buzzing around, gathering nectar. While most commercial blended varieties have an effect greater than or equal to that of sugar, some honeys have a low glycemic index. The range of glycemic index values from all the honeys that have been tested over the years runs from GI 32 up to GI 87. When the University of Sydney Glycemic Index Research Service tested pure wildflower (single floral) honeys—red gum, yellow box, ironbark, and others—produced by allowing bees access only to some types of gum trees (eucalypts), they found that these honeys all have a low glycemic index (GI 35 to 53). We would like to think it's possible that all pure wildflower honeys have only modest glycemic effects, but it is too early to say, as there hasn't been sufficient testing around the world. We do know that Romanian locust honey appears to have the lowest glycemic index value of all the honeys tested to date (GI 32).

Why all the differences in glycemic impact from one honey to another? To maintain a consistent flavor in commercial honeys, some of the more pungent components are removed. We suspect that these removed components are physiologically active and work to slow down absorption into the small intestine. For example, Australian wildflower honeys might contain alpha-glucosidase inhibitors that bees have extracted from the eucalypt flowers. We know that these potent inhibitors exist in many plants, and, indeed, some diabetic medications (e.g., acarbose) are based on pure forms of these inhibitors. In addition, it appears that the higher the fructose content, the lower the glycemic index is. Five German honeys with fructose content ranging from 38.5 to 43.5 percent not only had a low glycemic index (under GI 55), but also had a low insulinemic index (similar to the glycemic index, the insulin index is a relative ranking of the effect of 238 calories/1,000 kilojoules of food on blood insulin concentrations over a two-hour period).

Honey is one of the most adaptable sweeteners. People enjoy it as a spread, topping, and sweetener for hot or cold beverages. It is also a very popular ingredient in beer making. Honey is hygroscopic, meaning that it pulls moisture from the air, so when you bake a cake with honey, it tends to stay moist. Cooking with honey is delicious but can be tricky, as flavor and sweetness levels vary considerably depending on where the bees gathered their nectar. "Like wine and cheese, honey is a distillation of its immediate environment," says Australian food writer Kate McGhie, who shared these sweet pointers with us:

- "Honey is great for glazing roasted and baked foods; stir through hot liquids for a pick-me-up; drizzle over thin slices of cheese as a sweet-and-salty end to a meal; soothe winter colds with hot water, lemon juice, and a spoonful of eucalyptus honey; add to stir-fries with soy, crushed garlic, and grated ginger; or whip unsalted butter and runny honey to flavor vegetables or spread on toast.
- It can be dense or free-flowing, though most honey is heated and filtered, which makes it stay liquid. Untreated honeys

will crystallize, which does not affect the quality, but to make it liquid again, put the jar in a warm place for a while.

- Honey keeps baked products moist. But using all honey and no sugar in baking produces a chewy texture in cakes and biscuits. Add a pinch of baking soda (bicarbonate of soda) to counteract honey's natural acidity.
- A honey batter crisps and browns faster than a sugar batter. It also needs beating longer and more vigorously than sugar batter."

▶ HONEY AT A GLANCE

Nutritive

Sugars Fructose, glucose, sucrose, plus small amounts maltose, trehalose, turanose (varies depending on nectar source)

Sweetness relative to sucrose Equally sweet to about 50% sweeter

Calories 22 calories (94 kilojoules) per level teaspoon

Health Contains ▶FODMAPs; avoid giving to babies under 12 months

Why should you avoid giving honey to babies under 12 months?

▶**Honey** can become contaminated with the bacteria *clostridium botulinum*, and children under the age of 12 months are particularly sensitive to the toxin produced by the bacteria—botox (yes, the same one used in facial injections for anti-aging treatments).

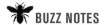 BUZZ NOTES

Honey Labeling—and Misleading Labeling

Winnie the Pooh had no problems when he wanted a jar of ▶**honey**. The jar very clearly said "HONEY" (or "HUNNY") and that is exactly what was in it. These days many jars on supermarket shelves say "honey" on the label, but what's inside is in fact a blend of honey with another sweetener such as ▶**corn syrup**. The honey has been adulterated and the product misbranded (i.e., labeled in a false and misleading way).

It's perfectly legal for producers and food companies to market honey blended with other sweeteners, but if they do (usually to cut costs), they are required to label it as a blend—e.g., "blend of honey and corn syrup" or "blend of corn syrup and honey" depending on which ingredient is predominant. If they don't, they can be prosecuted and fined by the appropriate food regulatory authorities. But of course, the regulatory authorities have to find the misbranded product first.

Honey standards and labeling requirements vary slightly from country to country. The international FAO/WHO Codex Alimentarius Standard requires that:

> Honey sold as such shall not have added to it any food ingredient, including food additives, nor shall any other additions be made other than honey. Honey shall not have any objectionable matter, flavour, aroma, or taint absorbed from foreign matter during its processing and storage. The honey shall not have begun to ferment or effervesce. No pollen or constituent particular to honey may be removed except where this is unavoidable in the removal of foreign inorganic or organic matter.[23]

US food regulations do not have a standard for honey based on the 2001 *Revised Codex Alimentarius Commission's Standard for Honey*. But, as in many countries, there is an ongoing problem of adulteration and misleading labeling, especially with imported honey. In an effort to clarify the rules regarding misbranding and adulteration for the food industry, the FDA issued a draft guidance for industry in April 2014. Food companies and other producers who add sweeteners to honey will have to alert consumers by labeling their products as a blend.

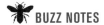 **BUZZ NOTES**

The Remarkable Honeybird

The Abyssins [Abyssinians] have many sorts of fowls both wild and tame . . . But amongst all their birds there is none more remarkable than the moroc, or honey-bird, which is furnished by nature with a peculiar instinct or faculty of discovering honey. They have here multitudes of bees of various kinds; some are tame, like ours, and form their combs in hives. Of the wild ones, some place their honey in hollow trees, others hide it in holes in the ground, which they cover so carefully, that though they are commonly in the highway, they are seldom found, unless by the moroc's help, which, when he has discovered any honey, repairs immediately to the road side, and when he sees a traveller, sings, and claps his wings, making many motions to invite him to follow him, and when he perceives him coming, flies before him from tree to tree, till he comes to the place where the bees have stored their treasure, and then begins to sing melodiously. The Abyssin takes the honey, without failing to leave part of it for the bird, to reward him for his information. This kind of honey I have often tasted, and do not find that it differs from the other sorts in anything but color; it is somewhat blacker. The great quantity of honey that is gathered, and a prodigious number of cows that is kept here, have often made me call Abyssinia a land of honey and butter.

—*A Voyage to Abyssinia*, by Father Jerónimo Lobo, a Portuguese Missionary (translated from the French by Samuel Johnson in 1789)[24]

HONEYDEW AND HONEYDEW HONEY

Not to be confused with the melon, sweet, sticky honeydew is plant sap that has been processed by aphids and other sap-sucking (psyllid) insects such as scale insects and whiteflies. It contains several sugars: ▶**sucrose**, ▶**glucose**, ▶**fructose**, and smaller amounts of ▶**maltose**, ▶**melezitose**, and ▶**fructomaltose**. The sap nourishes the aphids and other insects, and the honeydew they produce nourishes many other insects. Ants are particularly fond of it, and to ensure a regular supply, some will "herd" aphids, carrying them from plant to plant.

In Australia, honeydew has been a regular part of the Indigenous diet for thousands of years, especially in the form of *lerp* (a crystallized honeydew structure produced by larvae of psyllid insects as a protective cover). This is still a popular "bush tucker" treat for Indigenous children.

Although honeybees prefer nectar, they will sometimes collect honeydew in addition, and the resulting aromatic honeydew honey (also called forest honey, pine honey, fir honey, and beech honey) is as close as most of us will get to tasting honeydew itself. The best known is honeydew honey from Germany's Black Forest. Honeydew honeys typically have lower levels of glucose and fructose than flower honeys do, and higher levels of complex sugars (maltose, ▶**erlose**, and melezitose) due to the extra enzymatic action in the sap-sucking insect's gut.

▶ HONEYDEW AND HONEYDEW HONEY AT A GLANCE
Nutritive
Sugars Glucose, fructose, maltose, erlose, melezitose (Honeydew honey from New Zealand Beech)
Sweetness relative to sucrose Equally sweet
Calories 16 calories (67 kilojoules) per level teaspoon

HYDROGENATED STARCH HYDROLYSATE

Think of hydrogenated starch hydrolysate (HSH) as a broad group or family of ▶**polyol** (▶**sugar alcohol**) additives. They are used in processed foods (especially "sugar-free" products) as ▶**bulk sweeteners**, because they have a number of useful properties. In baked goods, for example, they help maintain moistness, preventing products from drying out; in sugar-free candy, they blend well with all kinds of flavors; and they do not crystallize.

They are made by the partial hydrolysis (meaning, breaking apart with water) of corn, potato, or wheat ▶**starch** into ▶**glucose** molecules or shorter glucose chains, which are then converted into sugar alcohols by a process called hydrogenation (adding hydrogen molecules). The end product is an ingredient (syrup or powder) composed of ▶**sorbitol**, ▶**maltitol**, and other ▶**oligo-** and ▶**polysaccharides**. They are typically between 25 to 50 percent as sweet as ▶**sucrose**, provide fewer calories per gram (3 as opposed to 4), and have little effect on ▶**blood glucose** levels because they are generally poorly absorbed (the body treats them more like a dietary ▶**fiber**).

Which HSH is which? It gets confusing for the consumer (and food label decoder), since the term is so broad. The names found on ingredients labels are generally based on the main component of the particular HSH. For example:

If the main component (50 percent of more) is sorbitol, they are called sorbitol syrups.

If the main component (50 percent of more) is maltitol, they are called maltitol syrups, maltitol solutions, or hydrogenated ▶**glucose syrups**.

If there is no main component, they are simply called hydrogenated starch hydrolysate.

The upside: like other polyols, they are "tooth friendly." The downside: They may have a laxative effect or cause gas or diarrhea if you consume them in large amounts. These products can pose a particular problem for children and adolescents due to their smaller body size. If you need to follow a low-▶**FODMAP** diet, avoid these and other polyols.

ICING SUGAR AND SOFT ICING MIXTURE

(▶confectioners' sugar; ▶powdered sugar)
This is another name for confectioners' sugar, a finely ground and sifted ▶**granulated sugar** (▶**sucrose**) with a smooth texture used for making icings; hence, the name. It is typically blended with 3 to 4 percent cornstarch to keep it free-flowing and prevent it from clumping.

INULIN

Inulin is an ingredient you will see increasingly often on food labels, as it is being used in conjunction with ▶**high-intensity sweeteners** to enhance flavor and replace sugar and other ▶**nutritive sweeteners** in sugar-free, sugar-reduced, or "diet" products such as chocolate, baked goods, breakfast cereals, cereal bars, yogurt, and beverages. We have also spotted it in ▶**organic** ▶**stevia** sweeteners, in which it provides both bulk and a prebiotic bonus; although we can't digest it, the healthy bacteria (like *Bifidobacteria* and *Lactobacilli*) in our large intestine just lap it up. It's not a sweetener per se; it's a ▶**fructan**, a type of soluble dietary ▶**fiber** found in ▶agave, artichokes, asparagus, bananas, carrots, ▶**chicory root**, garlic, Jerusalem artichokes, jicama, leeks, onions, wheat, and ▶**yacon**. The food industry's main sources of inulin are chicory root and Jerusalem artichoke.

In simple terms, a fructan is a chain of ▶**fructose** molecules joined together. Short-chain fructans are known as ▶**fructooligosaccharides** (also called ▶**oligofructose**) and are about 30 percent as sweet as ▶**granulated sugar** (▶**sucrose**); longer-chain fructans are known as inulins and are only about 10 percent as sweet as granulated sugar. You may see it referred to as a functional food because, like other soluble fibers, it has a prebiotic effect—good for digestive health.

However, it is not suitable for people who are following a low-▶**FODMAP** diet due to digestive problems such as irritable bowel syndrome (IBS).

INVERT SYRUP OR SUGAR

▶**Granulated sugar** is ▶**sucrose**, a ▶**disaccharide** consisting of ▶**glucose** and ▶**fructose** molecules that are joined together. If you heat sugar syrup for about thirty minutes with an acid such as cream of tartar or lemon juice, most of the sucrose will break down into separate glucose and fructose molecules. The technical term for this splitting is inversion, and the syrup you end up with is called invert syrup (or invert sugar, even though the final product is liquid, not crystals). Not all the sucrose splits: full invert syrup is about 90 percent separated glucose and fructose and 10 percent sucrose; medium is around 45 to 55 percent separated glucose and fructose and 45 to 55 percent sucrose.

Invert syrup is a clear liquid with a clean, slightly sweeter-than-sugar taste that is used in candies, fondant, jellies, sorbet, and ice cream because it helps control crystallization and gives the final product a smooth texture and creamy mouthfeel. You can buy it in specialty cake-decorating stores and online or make your own, following the process above. Although ▶**honey** is a natural source of invert sugar, it is not widely used as a substitute, since its distinctive flavor would change the taste of the recipe. ▶**Golden syrup** is an example of a medium inverted syrup.

▶ **INVERT SYRUP OR SUGAR AT A GLANCE (Full invert syrup)**
   Nutritive
   Sugars Glucose, fructose, sucrose
   Sweetness relative to sucrose About 20% sweeter
   Calories 16 calories (67 kilojoules) per level teaspoon

ISOMALT

Isomalt, a ▶**polyol** (sugar alcohol) derived from ▶**sugar beet**, is used as a sugar replacer in more than 1,800 products in over eighty countries, including the United States, the European Union, Japan, Australia, New Zealand, and many Eastern European, Asian, and South American countries. Its major role in the food and pharmaceutical industries is in sugar-free/"tooth-friendly" products such as sweets (hard candies, chocolate, and chewing gum), jams and spreads, ice creams and sorbets, chewable tablets, cough drops, throat lozenges, and nutritional supplements.

In addition, isomalt comes to the fore in sugar art; it is resistant to humidity, and chefs and cake decorators find it easy and quick to work with. If you see an elaborately decorated cake in a television advertisement or on a baking reality show such as *Ace of Cakes* or *The Cake Boss*, you can be pretty sure isomalt is playing a key role behind the scenes.

Developed by Beneo-Palatinit, isomalt is derived from ▶**sucrose**, but the process is more complicated than marketing phrases (such as "sugar born" or "the natural origin of this sugar replacer") suggest. To cut a long story short, the ▶**fructose** portion of sucrose is converted to equal amounts of ▶**sorbitol** and ▶**mannitol**. The ▶**glucose** portion is unchanged. Thus, isomalt is a mixture of two ▶**disaccharides**: glucose-sorbitol and glucose-mannitol.

As a bulk sweetener, crystalline isomalt looks very much like ▶**regular sugar** and for this reason is often combined in products with ▶**high-intensity sweeteners** (**HIS**) to provide texture and structure. It has half the calories of regular sugar (2 calories per gram compared with 4), and because it is very poorly absorbed (the body treats it as a dietary ▶**fiber**), it has virtually no effect on ▶**blood glucose** levels (GI 2). Like other polyols, it is considered "tooth friendly." The downside is its laxative effect if consumed in large quantities. Also, because it contains polyols, it is not suitable for those following a low-FODMAP diet.

Because it is used for making hard candies and pulled-sugar items, you will find isomalt crystals, as well as clear or colored nibs (precooked isomalt that can be melted in the microwave) in specialty cake decorating and sugar art stores and online.

▶ ISOMALT AT A GLANCE

Nutritive

Sugars Glucose, sorbitol, mannitol (Palatinose brand)

Sweetness relative to sucrose About 45–65% as sweet

Calories 8 calories (34 kilojoules) per level teaspoon

FDA approval GRAS status

EFSA Number E953

ADI Not specified

LTV 29 grams per meal (JEFCA)

Health Contains ▶FODMAPs

ISOMALTULOSE

Isomaltulose is a sugar naturally present in very small amounts in ▶honey and ▶sugarcane. Compared with ▶granulated sugar (▶sucrose), it has a significantly slower rate of digestion and absorption because the bond linking the ▶glucose and ▶fructose molecules in this ▶disaccharide is harder to break down: the glycemic index of ▶regular sugar is 65 (average); isomaltose is GI 32. It is also less likely to cause cavities than sucrose.

Palatinose™, the commercial version of isomaltulose, is manufactured from sucrose from ▶sugar beet. Developed as a "low glycemic" sweetener, it's marketed as a sucrose substitute to people with diabetes wanting to manage their ▶blood glucose levels, as well as to endurance athletes looking for sustained energy. It has also found a ready market with bodybuilders. It has been approved for use as a novel food (a nontraditional food that requires assessment to establish its safety before being introduced into the food supply) in Europe and Australia and has GRAS status in the United States.

It has the same number of calories per gram as sugar (4) but is only about half as sweet, so you need to use more to get the same level of sweetness, which, of course, ups the calorie and carb count. On a day-to-day basis, using it in place of regular sugar might help people with diabetes reduce the overall glycemic index of their diet. However, the results of a study published in *Diabetes Care* in 2012 reported that a group of people with type 2 diabetes who replaced sugar with isomaltulose for twelve weeks in their beverages and as toppings for foods didn't achieve better blood glucose control. (This was assessed by a glycated hemoglobin test—sometimes abbreviated as HbA1c—a lab test that shows the average level of blood glucose over the previous three months and shows how well a person is managing his or her diabetes). It was, however, associated with lower triglyceride levels.[25]

You can buy Palatinose™ online and in health food stores that sell nutrition and bodybuilding supplements. The food and beverage industry uses it in sports and fitness drinks, dairy products, energy and nutrition bars, baked goods, meal replacements, supplements and "nutraceuticals," and tabletop sweeteners.

▶ ISOMALTULOSE AT A GLANCE

Nutritive

Sugars Glucose, fructose (Palatinose™ brand)

Sweetness relative to sucrose About 60% as sweet

FDA approval GRAS status

Calories 16 calories (67 kilojoules) per level teaspoon

J

JAGGERY

(▸*gur*)

Jaggery is a traditional sugar made throughout Asia by concentrating freshly extracted ▸**cane juice** or the sap of various ▸**palms**. Technically, it is a ▸**raw**, ▸**non-centrifugal sugar**. This kind of sugar has numerous names, but jaggery is probably the most commonly used, certainly in India, Africa, and Myanmar (Burma). It is also called *gur* (in India and Pakistan), *desi* (in Pakistan), *hakuru* (in Sri Lanka), and ▸**kokuto** (in Okinawa). Whatever the name, it is essentially the same partially refined product as ▸**panela**, the non-centrifugal sugar made on family farms in small ▸**sugarcane** mills (*trapiches*) throughout Latin America and the Caribbean. In India, its production is an important cottage industry that provides jobs and can be set up with minimal investment of capital. India produces more than 70 percent of the world's jaggery—about 7 million tons a year—employing around 2.5 million people.

In South Asia, jaggery is much more than a sweetener. It is considered to be therapeutic, and, in Ayurveda, it is used as a base material to prepare medicines for certain ailments. Because it retains many of the minerals (particularly calcium, phosphorous, and iron) that are lost in refining ▸**white sugar**, it is thought to be a healthier choice. In very poor, rural areas where millions of people are malnourished and/or undernourished, it is possible that consuming jaggery improves the nutritional quality of an individual's diet by providing micronutrients as well as calories (energy). However, for those in well-nourished (and overnourished) societies, the amounts of micronutrients present are too minute to count toward anyone's recommended daily intake in an appreciable way, so don't use them as an excuse to add an extra spoonful. It's still sugar (mostly ▸**sucrose**) and comes with the same calories you would get from ▸**granulated**

sugar. Therefore, like all ▶**nutritive sweeteners**, it might contribute to weight gain, and it will elevate ▶**blood glucose** levels in people with diabetes when consumed in excessive amounts.

Solid jaggery, which is dense and sticky, ranges in color from golden yellow to dark brown and comes in a wide variety of shapes and sizes: rough cylinders, cones, cubes, blocks, and balls ranging in size from that of a marble to a coconut. Granular and liquid (▶**kakvi**) jaggery are also available. If buying it from specialty Asian or Indian produce stores or online, you are most likely to find blocks or cones. The label should tell you whether it is cane or palm jaggery.

With a toffee/caramellike aroma and a flavor somewhere between ▶**brown sugar** and ▶**molasses**, it is perfect for adding to desserts such as spicy coconut custard (*vattalappam*) and for sweetening a cup of chai. But you will also find it added to savory dishes to enhance flavors. Don't be surprised to see a little jaggery in the ingredients list for a vegetable curry or spicy *sambar*. It also makes its way into lentil soups (*dal*) to balance the spicy, salty, and sour tastes. It can be hard to measure out a level teaspoon, tablespoon, or cup of jaggery, so recipe writers often suggest you weigh it for accuracy. To use, simply chop or grate as per the recipe's requirements.

▶ **JAGGERY AT A GLANCE**
   Nutritive
   Sugars Sucrose, glucose, fructose
   Sweetness relative to sucrose Equally sweet
   Calories 16 calories (67 kilojoules) per level teaspoon

JAM SETTING SUGAR

Jam setting sugar is a ▶**granulated sugar** blend specifically formulated to help get a good set when making jams and preserves with fruits low in pectin (see Buzz Notes on page 100). It contains everything the home preserver needs to get the set right. CSR Jam Setting Sugar, for example, lists as its ingredients: Sugar (98%), Gelling Agent (Pectin) (0.7%), Acidity Regulator (Citric Acid), Vegetable Oil.

▶ **JAM SETTING SUGAR AT A GLANCE**
   Nutritive
   Sugars Sucrose
   Sweetness relative to sucrose Equally sweet
   Calories 16 calories (67 kilojoules) per level teaspoon

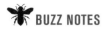

BUZZ NOTES
Pectin

To achieve a good set with jams, jellies, preserves, and marmalades, you need pectin combined with exactly the right amount of sugar and fruit. Pectin, a type of ▶**fiber** found in the cell walls of plants, gives fruit its structure and firmness. French chemist Henri Braconnot first isolated pectin in 1825. It is found naturally in fruit and vegetables, but to a greater or lesser extent, which is why some fruits set without added pectin, and others don't. A crunchy apple is rich in pectin; a squishy strawberry has far less. Here is a quick guide to pectin highs and lows:

- Higher-pectin fruits include apples and most citrus fruits (oranges, lemons, limes, kumquats, etc.). These fruits can be used alone (with or without ▶**preserving sugar**) or added to lower-pectin fruits and berries to ensure a good set.
- Moderate and lower-pectin fruits include berries, (strawberries, raspberries, blackberries, blueberries, etc.), stone fruits (plums, apricots, peaches, nectarines, etc.), figs, and rhubarb. If you don't want to mix fruits, you can use a commercial pectin (it is available in dried or liquid form) or a ▶**jam setting sugar**.

JAPANESE BLACK SUGAR

This is the traditional ▶**non-centrifugal** ▶**cane sugar** (▶**sucrose**) made in Okinawa. Look for it in specialty Japanese or Asian produce stores or online, or replace it with ▶**muscovado** or ▶**brown sugar** in recipes. *See also* ▶**black sugar**

KAKVI JAGGERY

Sweet, syrupy *kakvi* or *kakavi* is the cane syrup that is produced as a by-product of ▶**jaggery** production. It is not widely available. But in some parts of rural India, it is used instead of jaggery for sweetening curries, desserts, and beverages.

KOKUTO

You will find Okinawa's traditional ▶**non-centrifugal sugar** in specialty Japanese or Asian produce stores or online; in recipes, you can replace it with ▶**muscovado** or ▶**brown sugar**.

See also ▶**black sugar**

L

LACTITOL

Lactitol is a ▶**polyol** (sugar alcohol) manufactured by reducing the ▶**glucose** part of the ▶**disaccharide** ▶**lactose**. As a reduced-calorie ▶**bulk sweetener** with a "sugar-like" taste, it's widely used by the food industry on its own or blended with other sweeteners in "diet" versions of cookies, candy, ice cream, chewing gum, and chocolate. It is also used in laxative preparations for the prevention and/or treatment of constipation. Unlike other sugar alcohols, such as ▶**erythritol** or ▶**xylitol**, it's not available as a consumer product for home cooking or use as a tabletop sweetener.

The upside: It has just over half the calories of ▶**granulated sugar** (2.4 calories per gram, compared with 4), and because it is very poorly absorbed by the body and only partly metabolized, it has virtually no effect on ▶**blood glucose** levels and can be safely consumed by people who are lactose intolerant. In addition, like other polyols, it does not promote cavities. However, the downside, as with many other polyols, is its laxative effect if consumed in large quantities.

▶ **LACTITOL AT A GLANCE**

Nutritive

Sugars Lactitol

Sweetness relative to sucrose About 30–40% as sweet

Calories 2.4 calories (10 kilojoules) per level teaspoon (based on US 2; Europe 2.4 calories per gram for labeling purposes)

FDA approval GRAS status

EFSA Number E966

ADI Not specified

LTV 24–50 grams per meal (JEFCA)

Health Contains ▶**FODMAPs**

LACTOSE

Lactose, or milk sugar, is a ▶**disaccharide** (made of ▶**galactose** and ▶**glucose** molecules) about half as sweet as ▶**granulated sugar** (▶**sucrose**). It is the primary ▶**carbohydrate** in all mammals' milk—cow, goat, sheep, buffalo, camel, and human—and thus is part of the total nutritional package containing all the proteins, fats, vitamins, and carbohydrates that babies (human and animal) need to grow and thrive and fight infection. Human breast milk has the highest lactose concentrations of any mammal's, with around 8 grams per half cup at peak lactation—almost double that of cows' milk.

Lactose needs to be broken down into its component sugars, glucose and galactose, before the body can use it. Lactase—a lactose-breaking, genetically controlled enzyme located in the small intestine—does this for us. Until we are three or four years of age, most of us have sufficient lactase to digest lactose. After this, lactase production virtually grinds to halt in 65 percent of us (as well as in animals, including dogs, cats, rats, mice, etc.).

The ability to digest milk after early childhood changed for some groups of humans about ten thousand years ago when they settled down, became farmers and herders, and added milk from their domesticated animals to their diet. Within a thousand years or so of their doing so, a genetic mutation allowed many of them to keep producing lactase beyond childhood, thus enabling them to continue digesting the lactose in milk. Research on DNA from skeleton remains in central Europe found that about 80 percent of people in the area had the genetic mutation for tolerating lactose about seven thousand years ago, and over time, the mutation became dominant in parts of Europe through to northern India. It is thought that the same genetic mutation occurred independently in North Africa and the Middle East when the camel became domesticated and camel milk became part of the diet. Marlene Zuk, PhD, author of *Paleofantasy*, describes adults' ability to digest milk as the "poster child" for rapid evolution in humans. Today, it is estimated that around 35 percent of people carry the mutation and can digest milk and milk products over their lifetime.

Even if you are lactose intolerant, you can enjoy yogurt. This is because the microorganisms added to milk to make yogurt are active in digesting lactose—in other words, the "bugs" help do the job of lactose digestion for you. Alternatively, you can find lactose-free dairy foods in your local supermarket; the lactose has been broken down to glucose and galactose by the addition of the enzyme lactase to the product. You can also buy pure lactase (e.g., Lactaid® pills) and take it with dairy foods.

Lactose intolerance in infants (congenital lactase deficiency), caused by mutations in the LCT gene, brings about a severely impaired ability to digest the lactose in breast milk or formula, so as soon as it is identified, babies are fed lactose-free formula. Congenital lactase deficiency is not the same as the acquired lactase deficiency that occurs in many humans after weaning.

Lactose has the same number of calories and carbohydrates per gram as sucrose but a low glycemic index (GI 46). This is because, once absorbed, the galactose is mainly metabolized in the liver and, thus, has very little effect on ▶**blood glucose** levels. The remaining sugar, glucose, which has a high glycemic index (GI 100), is present in small amounts that do not cause a spike in blood glucose levels.

Lactose is naturally found in milk, yogurt, and many, but not all, dairy foods. The richest sources are whey and milk powder. Hard cheeses (such as cheddar, Gruyère, Parmesan, pecorino, and Swiss) are not a source of lactose, as they have almost no carbohydrates; they drain away in the whey. Pure lactose is rarely added to foods or beverages as an ingredient, but it can, of course, be found in milk-based ingredients that are commonly added to foods. The notable exception is infant formula, where it is needed to match the composition of human milk. It is also used in pharmaceutical products as filler because it is inexpensive and easy to compress.

▶ LACTOSE AT A GLANCE

Nutritive

Sugars Galactose, glucose

Sweetness relative to sucrose About 40% as sweet

Calories 16 calories (67 kilojoules) per level teaspoon

Health Contains lactose

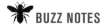 **BUZZ NOTES**

Breast Milk: The Perfect Sweet Package for Babies

▶**Lactose** is an ideal example of our philosophy that if you want to add a little sweetness to your life, it's best to add it to healthy foods that bring something to the table apart from calories. Mother Nature showed us the way. The appealing sweetness of the sugar lactose in breast milk—the food Mother Nature designed for human babies—is part of a nutritional package that contains an amazing collection of protective goodies unique to human milk. Dr. Jennie Brand-Miller lists these "protective factors" in *The Low GI Eating Plan for an Optimal Pregnancy*. They include:

- ▶**Carbohydrates** that prevent pathogens from attaching to body surfaces
- Sugars that promote the growth of beneficial bacteria in the lower part of the digestive tract
- Antibodies known as immunoglobulins (IgA and IgG) that prevent binding and multiplication of pathogens
- Anti-inflammatory agents
- Antioxidants
- White blood cells
- Lactoferrin, a protein that binds iron and inhibits "bugs" that need iron for their growth
- Lysosyme, an enzyme that attacks pathogens
- Antivirals and other agents that prevent infections

LEVULOSE

Just as ▶**dextrose** (meaning "right turning") is another chemical term for ▶**glucose**; *levulose* (meaning "left turning,") is another term for ▶**fructose**, or fruit sugar (because a solution of fructose in water rotates the plane of polarized light to the left).

LICORICE

Licorice comes from the long, thick root of the licorice plant (*Glycyrrhiza glabra*, which means "sweet root"). Most people think of it not as a sweetener but as an aromatic, adding color and flavor to candies and some beers. Nonetheless, ▶**glycyrrhizin**, or glycyrrhizinic acid, is a sweet-tasting food additive extracted from the licorice root that is about 50 to 100 times sweeter than ▶**granulated sugar** (▶**sucrose**).

LOGICANE® SUGAR AND SOFT ICING MIXTURE

LoGiCane® is the brand name for low-GI ▶**cane sugar** (▶**sucrose**) and ▶**confectioners' sugar.** These products are equivalent to regular

▶granulated sugar and regular confectioners' sugar, but because of the innovative manufacturing process (the sugar is sprayed with ▶molasses extract, a natural by-product of sugarcane manufacture), they retain most of the nutrients from ▶sugarcane, such as minerals and antioxidant polyphenols, and they have a low glycemic index (GI 54), which means that ▶blood glucose levels will rise at a slower rate than from regular granulated sugar. LoGiCane® products are currently available only in Australia and New Zealand, although we understand there are plans to make them available elsewhere. *See also* ▶raw sugar

▶ LOGICANE SUGAR AND SOFT ICING MIXTURE AT A GLANCE

Nutritive

Sugars Sucrose (LoGiCane sugar brand)

Sweetness relative to sucrose Equally sweet

Calories 16 calories (67 kilojoules) per level teaspoon

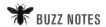 BUZZ NOTES

Polyphenols

LoGiCane was developed by Horizon Science, an R&D technology company that focuses primarily on developing innovative polyphenol-enhanced products derived from ▶sugarcane waste streams; it sprays all-natural ▶molasses extract onto ▶raw sugar, which decreases the absorption of ▶monosaccharides in the small intestine. The company's research to date has identified a range of phytochemicals in molasses capable of positively changing body composition.

LUCUMA POWDER

Lucuma powder, a mildly sweet flavoring sold in health and ▶organic stores and online, is also marketed as a replacement sweetener. Native to Peru, lucuma (*Pouteria lucuma*) is a starchy, nutritious fruit from the Sapotaceae family with dryish (some describe it as "mealy") flesh that's rich in beta-carotene and ▶fiber. It can be eaten ripe, but more typically the pulp is added to drinks, pies, and desserts or is dried and milled into a fine powder (flour) that keeps well; blends easily into ice creams, yogurts, and smoothies; and is added to chocolate, baked goods, and desserts.

Being very much the new kid on the alternative-sweetener block, lucuma powder has its share of "superfood" claims but no solid nutritional data or peer-reviewed research on its health benefits. It certainly hasn't made it into the USDA National Nutrient Database for Standard Reference. We checked the nutrition-facts panels on a number of brands and found that most (but not all) agree that 1 tablespoon of lucuma powder has 60 calories and 13 grams total ▶**carbohydrates**, which includes 2 grams of sugars and 11 grams of ▶**starch**.

Because it is low in sugars, it is often marketed as "diabetic friendly." We have even seen claims that it has a low glycemic index. The jury is still out on that, as its glycemic index hasn't been tested following the internationally standardized method. We would guess that its glycemic index is more likely to be moderate, possibly similar to that of other orange-fleshed, starchy fruits and vegetables from South America, such as sweet potato (*Ipomoea batatas)*. Until it has been tested, if you need to manage your ▶**blood glucose** levels, know that 1 tablespoon lucuma powder is equal to about one 15-gram carbohydrate exchange. Remember that foods labeled as "reduced sugar" may still contain carbohydrates. Sugar is only one type of carbohydrate that affects blood glucose levels. Starch is the other.

The simplest way to add lucuma to your day as an alternative to sugar or other sweeteners is to add the powder to plain yogurt or a smoothie for a delicate caramel flavor. If you want to replace all or part of the sugar in desserts and baking, check similar recipes on the suppliers' websites for an idea of how much to use when substituting.

▶ **LUCUMA POWDER AT A GLANCE**

Nutritive

Sugars Glucose, fructose, sucrose

Sweetness relative to sucrose Much less sweet

Calories 20 calories (84 kilojoules) per level teaspoon

LUO HAN GUO

(lo han guo; ▶*monk fruit)*

This is another name for monk fruit (*Siraitia grosvenorii*). The process for extracting the active ingredient (a ▶**high-intensity sugar** called a ▶**mogroside**, technically classified as triterpene glucosides) from the fruit was patented by Procter & Gamble in 1995. Monk fruit has GRAS status in the United States as a sweetener. It is 200 to 400 times sweeter than regular ▶**granulated sugar**.

MABINLIN

Mabinlin is a ▶**protein** that is derived from the sweet-tasting seeds of mabinlang (*Capparis masaikai*), a fruit the size of a tennis ball and native to China's Yunnan province. The seeds have long been chewed as a snack and used in traditional Chinese medicine. It is, in fact, a family of sweet proteins (four have been isolated so far: mabinlin-1, -2, -3, -4) that were first identified in 1993 and are about 100 to 400 times sweeter than ▶**sucrose**. The sweetest is mabinlin-2. As a protein, it provides 4 calories per gram, but since such a minute amount of the active ingredient is required to sweeten, it is considered to be a ▶**nonnutritive sweetener**. It does not have regulatory approval for use as a food additive.

▶ **MABINLIN AT A GLANCE**

Nutritive

Sweetness relative to sucrose About 100–400 times sweeter

Calories 4 calories (17 kilojoules) per gram

FDA approval No

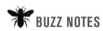 **BUZZ NOTES**

Not Yet on the Shelf but Maybe on the Radar

▶**Mabinlin**, ▶**monatin**, and ▶**monellin**: Not one of these three sweet ▶**proteins** derived from plants has made it to market yet. You won't find them in any foods or drinks as ▶**nonnutritive sweeteners**, as, at the time of writing, for a wide range of logistical, taste, and performance reasons, they have not yet been commercialized, and they do not have regulatory approval for use as food additives in any country. Of course, in their homelands the actual fruits and roots that the additives are extracted from have been enjoyed by the locals for hundreds (possibly thousands) of years.

MALT

Malt (and malting) dates back several thousand years to the Neolithic Revolution, when our nomadic hunter-gatherer forebears settled down and became farmers, growing grain and domesticating sheep, goats, and cattle. Malting is the process they discovered, probably by chance, that converted the largely indigestible ▶**starch** in their staple grains (barley, rice, sorghum, and wheat) into a digestible product, which they could store and use in a variety of ways, such as milling it to make flour, fermenting it to make beer, or mashing it with water and concentrating it to make a sweetener.

Malting itself is simply the process of inducing a grain to partially germinate by steeping it in water until tiny rootlets sprout through the seed coating. As this happens, growth hormones (gibberellins) kick-start the enzyme amylase to convert the grain's stored starch into sugars that will feed the growing plant. But, of course, the plant doesn't grow, because at this point the grain is dried in a kiln, halting the germination process. To make syrup, malted grains are mashed with water and cooked. This reactivates the enzymes that convert the starches to sugars. The liquid is then drained and concentrated to produce a malt syrup that is about 45 percent ▶**maltose**, 3 percent ▶**glucose**, and 52 percent ▶**maltotriose**.

See also ▶**barley malt syrup**; ▶**rice syrup**

Does a spoonful of sugar really help the medicine go down?

Mary Poppins was right: it really does. Throughout much of the twentieth century, a little malt extract in the mixture helped millions of children down their nasty-tasting, bone-building, rickets-preventing dose of cod liver oil, with its vitamins D and A, and omega-3 fatty acids. These days, the sweetener in medicines from cough syrups to chewable multivitamin tablets is more likely to be an artificial one, such as ▶**saccharin** or a ▶**sorbitol** and ▶**aspartame** blend. Who's for ▶**malt**?

MALTITOL

Maltitol, manufactured from ▶**maltose**, is one of the sweetest ▶**polyols** (▶**sugar alcohols**): it's 75 to 90 percent as sweet as ▶**sucrose**. It is available as syrup or crystallized to a powder. The food industry adds it to "diet" foods to replace sugar (sucrose), as it provides equivalent bulk, texture, and preservative benefits, and to replace fat, as it gives a creamy texture to food. You will find it in the ingredients lists for diet or sugar-free products such as hard candies, chewing gum, cough drops, chocolate, baked goods, and ice cream.

As a ▶**bulk sweetener**, crystalline maltitol looks very much like ▶**granulated sugar**, but it has fewer calories (about 3 calories per gram compared with 4), and because it is poorly absorbed (the body treats it more like a dietary ▶**fiber**), it has virtually no effect on ▶**blood glucose** levels (GI 26). Like most other polyols, it is considered "tooth friendly," but it may have a laxative effect.

▶ MALTITOL AT A GLANCE

Nutritive

Sugars Maltitol

Sweetness relative to sucrose About 75–90% as sweet

Calories 2.4 calories (10 kilojoules) per level teaspoon (based on US 1.6; EU 2.4; ANZ 3.1 calories per gram for labeling purposes)

FDA approval GRAS status

EFSA Number E965

ADI Not specified

LTV 60 grams per meal (JEFCA)

Health Contains ▶**FODMAPs**

MALTODEXTRIN

Think of maltodextrin (modified food ▶**starch**) as a family group, not as an individual ingredient. Maltodextrins are ▶**carbohydrates**: chains of ▶**glucose** molecules ranging from three to nine glucose units long. They are produced by processing corn (maize), potato, rice, tapioca, or wheat to break down the starch. As they are flavorless and only moderately sweet, they are commonly added to processed foods to provide bulk and texture and to help blend ingredients together. You will also find them in the single-serving, tabletop packets of some alternative sweeteners and in pharmaceuticals. Maltodextrin is listed in the FDA's Code of Federal Regulations (CFR) as a GRAS additive.

 Is maltodextrin gluten-free?

In the United States and Canada, ▶**maltodextrins** are most often made from corn, potato, or rice; in Europe, Australia, and New Zealand, wheat is widely used. It seems to be generally accepted that the source may not matter, since the original grain or starchy vegetable is highly processed to remove all the gluten-containing protein. However, dietitian Kate Marsh, PhD, author of *Low GI Gluten-Free Cooking*, always recommends that people with celiac disease avoid maltodextrin derived from wheat. "There is a possibility it may contain small amounts of gluten," she told us. "Wheat will appear on the label when it has been used to make maltodextrin. If you have celiac disease and are concerned about a particular product, your local celiac society should be able to help. Alternatively, check with your doctor or dietitian."

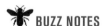 BUZZ NOTES
Beyond Maltodextrins: Sugar to Refined Starches

When there are ten or more linked ▶**glucose** molecules, it is no longer a ▶**maltodextrin**; it is now a ▶**polysaccharide,** technically called a ▶**starch** or refined starch.

With the heated debate about sugar, particularly added sugar (see page 211) and ▶**fructose**, it's easy to forget that sugars only make up around half of the ▶**carbohydrates** in the foods we eat. Everyone seems to have forgotten about the other form of carbohydrates we consume: starches (formerly known as complex carbohydrates). There is nothing inherently wrong with starch, which appears in traditional, nutrient-rich foods such as root vegetables, legumes, cracked wheat, brown rice, pearl barley, quinoa, and rolled oats. However, *refined* starches, such as cornstarch, may be worth more scrutiny than they've received to date.

First of all, most consumers don't realize that added starches are in many of the processed foods they buy. They seem to be "invisible." It's easy to understand why:

- They are not listed in the nutrition information/nutrition facts panel on foods.
- Their names are often unpronounceable, such as acetylated distarch phosphate (or food additive code number 1414, if you prefer).

Second, why does it matter? Refined starches contain essentially the same amount of calories (kilojoules) and total carbohydrates as refined sugars and, without fortification, are just as devoid of ►**fiber**, vitamins, and minerals. They also have a high glycemic index. In a nutshell, refined starches can be as detrimental to our health as refined sugar.

The modified food starches are E coded according to the International Numbering System (INS) for Food Additives:

1400 Dextrin roasted starch
1401 Acid-treated starch
1402 Alkaline-treated starch
1403 Bleached starch
1404 Oxidized starch
1405 Starches, enzyme treated
1410 Monostarch phosphate
1412 Distarch phosphate
1413 Phosphated distarch phosphate
1414 Acetylated distarch phosphate
1420 Starch acetate
1422 Acetylated distarch adipate
1440 Hydroxypropyl starch
1442 Hydroxypropyl distarch phosphate
1443 Hydroxypropyl distarch glycerol
1450 Starch sodium octenyl succinate
1451 Acetylated oxidized starch

How high is the GI of these refined starches relative to regular sugars?

It would be good to be able to provide specific numbers, but we can't, because unlike sugars (which you can ask people to consume for glycemic index testing), you cannot eat raw starch.

MALTOSE OR MALT SUGAR

Maltose, a ▶**disaccharide**, has a mild taste and is about 30 to 50 percent as sweet as ▶**granulated sugar** (▶**sucrose**). Made up of two ▶**glucose** molecules bound together, it is found in germinating grains such as barley, as well as in ▶**malt** and malted foods and beverages. It has one of the highest glycemic indexes of all foods tested to date (GI 105). As a sugar, it is used in bread making and beer brewing and added to processed foods to extend their shelf life. It is the main sugar in ▶**barley malt**, ▶**corn syrup**, and ▶**rice syrup**. On its own, it is not a consumer product, so you won't find it on the supermarket shelf.

▶ **MALTOSE OR MALT SUGAR AT A GLANCE**
   Nutritive
   Sugars Maltose
   Sweetness relative to sucrose About 30–50% as sweet
   Calories 16 calories (67 kilojoules) per level teaspoon

MALTOTRIOSE

When two single-sugar ▶**glucose** molecules are joined together, you get the ▶**disaccharide** ▶**maltose**. Add a third unit of ▶**glucose**, and you have the trisaccharide maltotriose, which is technically a ▶**maltodextrin**. Foods and beverages containing maltotriose include ▶**malt** syrup or extract and ▶**rice syrup**.

MANNITOL

Mannitol, a ▶**polyol** (▶**sugar alcohol**), has been used as a sugar replacer for over sixty years. Originally isolated from secretions of the flowering, or manna, ash (*Fraxinus ornus*), the white crystalline powder is now generally manufactured from ▶**fructose** or, in China, from seaweed. It is used by the food and pharmaceutical industries in sugar-free products such as chewing gum and chewy sweets, and in chewy tablets. It also has a number of medicinal applications.

It has about half the calories of ▶**granulated sugar** (▶**sucrose**)—approximately 2 calories per gram compared with 4—and because it is poorly absorbed (the body treats it like a dietary ▶**fiber**), it has virtually no effect on ▶**blood glucose** levels. Like most polyols, it is considered "tooth friendly" but may have a laxative effect if consumed in large quantities.

▶ **MANNITOL AT A GLANCE**

Nutritive

Sugars Mannitol

Sweetness relative to sucrose About 50–70% as sweet

Calories 2.2 calories (7 kilojoules) per level teaspoon (based on US 1.6; EU 2.4; ANZ 2.2 calories per gram for labeling purposes)

FDA approval Yes

EFSA Number E421

ADI Not specified

LTV 10–20 grams per meal (JEFCA)

Health Contains ▶FODMAPs

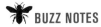 **BUZZ NOTES**

Manna from Plants

Manna is a term that has long been used to describe the mysterious sweet substances that appear in a wide range of plants. But it doesn't have a precise meaning at all. In the plant world, it's associated with seasonal attack by scale insects, but it's unclear whether manna is a gummy sap the plant exudes as a result of being attacked, or whether it is more like ▶**honeydew**, something the insect secretes and leaves behind. Charles Perry describes two of the mannas that have had importance as food in *The Oxford Companion to Food* this way:

> The best known is tamarisk manna, a white honey-like substance which appears in the desert tree *Tamarix mannifera* when infested by insects such as *Coccus manniparus*. This manna is known in Arabic as *mann*, in Persian as *taranjabin* (literally fresh honey because unlike bees' honey it is not enclosed in a comb but drips off the plant in hot weather). . . . By the time tamarisk manna enters commerce it is a grey sticky mass about 10% of which is glucose and fructose, the remainder being sucrose and several other non-reducing sugars plus inedible residue. . . . The second important manna appears on two spiny-branched shrubs known as camel's thorn, *Alhagi maurorum* and *A. Pseudalhagi*. It dries readily and is harvested by shaking the branches of the shrub over cloth. . . . Camel's thorn manna is primarily sucrose.[26]

MAPLE SYRUP AND SUGAR

We aren't the only species with a sweet tooth. The red squirrel *(Tamiasciurus hudsonicus)* has one, too. Biologist and author of the bestselling *Winter World: The Ingenuity of Animal Survival* Bernd Heinrich reported on their "sugaring behavior" in *Journal of Mammalogy* (1992) after watching them systematically tapping and harvesting syrup from sugar maples *(Acer saccharum)* in western Maine.[27] "Each tap," he writes, "consisted of a single pair of chisel-like grooves of an apparent single bite that punctured the tree to the sap-bearing xylem. The dripping dilute sap was not harvested. Instead the squirrels came back later and selectively visited the trees that had been punctured after most of the water from the sap had evaporated." Talk about emotional intelligence and the ability to delay gratification!

Since the red squirrel has inhabited the northeastern forests much longer than people have, there could well be something in the traditional story the Iroquois tell about the bright-eyed boy who saw a red squirrel biting a maple and later enjoying its sugary bark and so followed suit. The indigenous people of eastern North America were certainly making maple syrup long before the first European explorers arrived and established colonies, and they shared their sugaring techniques with the settlers. With the tax on sugar and consequent high price, maple sugar was a desirable and affordable alternative. Right up to the latter part of the nineteenth century, maple sugar was the primary product of sugaring (hence, the term). With the end of the tax and the advent of cheap ▶**cane sugar**, the maple sugar industry turned its focus to syrup, which is now found in domestic and restaurant kitchens around the world.

Syrup production is temperature sensitive. Maple trees' clear, slightly sweet, watery sap, which contains about 2 percent sugar, only flows from the tree's roots to its branches as winter gives way to spring and daytime temperatures climb above 40°F/4°C, falling below freezing (32°F/0°C) at night. The season is short: around four to six weeks. Once buds begin to form on the trees and the nights grow warmer, it is over. Although syrup-making technology has changed over time, the basic process is essentially the same. The sap is boiled down to evaporate the water and produce syrup. It takes about 40 to 50 gallons of sap to produce a gallon of syrup. The final product is about one-third water and two-thirds sugars (about 62 percent ▶**sucrose** with small amounts of ▶**glucose** and ▶**fructose**). Maple syrup has a low glycemic index (GI 54), making it a sweet topping alternative for people who need to manage their ▶**blood glucose** levels.

Pure, 100 percent maple syrup has a truly distinctive flavor, the hows and whys of which not even food scientists who specialize in taste, flavor, and aroma have been able fully explain. In addition, not all maple syrups are created equal. Flavors vary significantly from producer to producer, year to year, and time of season in which the sap was harvested. The final product is graded according to its translucency, because the color is the best guide to flavor and use. The table shows the current USDA grades and the new, more descriptive labeling system with four grades (B disappears) designed to make life simpler for consumers. This was rolled out voluntarily in Vermont in 2014 and will become mandatory in 2015.

CURRENT USDA GRADES	NEW VERMONT LABELING GRADES	CANADIAN GRADES
Grade A Light Amber	Grade A Golden Color/Delicate Taste	No. 1 Extra Light
Grade A Medium Amber	Grade A Amber Color/Rich Taste	No. 1 Light
Grade A Dark Amber	Grade A Dark Color/Robust Taste	No. 2 Medium
Grade B	Grade A Dark Color/Robust Taste	
Grade C Commercial Grade	Grade A Very Dark/Strong Taste	No. 3 Dark

Perhaps best known for being drizzled over pancakes, waffles, French toast, or oatmeal, maple syrup can also be swirled through plain yogurt or used in classic vinaigrettes and other dressings or to bring natural sweetness and depth to baking, glazing roasted vegetables, and flavoring bacon and ham.

Avoid the cheaper maple-flavored syrups—they aren't in the same culinary league, and the predominant sugar isn't sucrose. As these products are typically ▶**corn syrup** with a dash of maple syrup (or extract) for flavor, the sugar they contain will be high-GI glucose.

▶ MAPLE SYRUP AND SUGAR AT A GLANCE
Nutritive

Sugars Sucrose, glucose, fructose

Sweetness relative to sucrose About 90% as sweet

Calories 14 calories (61 kilojoules) per level teaspoon

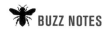 **BUZZ NOTES**

Maple Sugaring Without Metal or Fire

Colonel James Smith described this "remarkable occurrence" in 1799:

> Shortly after we came to this place, the squaws began to make sugar. We had no large kettles with us this year, and they made the frost, in some measure, supply the place of fire, in making sugar. Their large bark vessels, for holding the stock-water, they made broad and shallow; and as the weather is very cold here, it frequently freezes at night in sugar time; and the ice they break and cast out of the vessels. I asked them if they were not throwing away the sugar? They said no; it was water they were casting away, sugar did not freeze, and there was scarcely any in that ice. They said I might try the experiment, and boil some of it, and see what I would get. I never did try it; but I observed that after several times freezing, the water that remained in the vessel, changed its color and became brown and very sweet.[28]

 What's maple water?

Maple water is a refreshing drink straight from the tree when the sap is running in maple country, and not just in the United States and Canada. In South Korea, drinking maple sap (*gorosoe*) is a springtime ritual with festivals and sap-drinking contests. Until recently, maple water had a very limited season, as it could only be harvested during a narrow, six-week window. According to the manufacturer of KiKi Maple Sweet Water®, "The sap is frozen to maintain its healthful benefits and maximize its fresh shelf life. At a local bottling plant, a hot fill process, with the liquid heated to just below 96 degrees Celsius, ensures that the drink remains below pasteurization temperature to preserve its purity, highlight the flavor and maintain healthful benefits. The product is then shipped, stored, and served chilled."

Jennie Brand-Miller described maple water this way in *GI News*:

> KiKi has about 60 calories (250 kilojoules) per 10 fluid ounce (300 ml) serving. Its light maple sweetness comes from the 2 to 3 percent concentration of sugars in the sap, but that still gives you around 15 grams or 3 teaspoons of sugar (sucrose, glucose, and fructose) in a serving. There are claims that it has a low GI value, but there is no actual GI for it on the

[Q&A continues]

[*continued* from page 117]

international database, as it has not been glycemic index tested (or the results have not been published). We assume the present claim is based on the GI for maple syrup (GI 54). It would be good to see it properly tested. If it is only 2 to 3 percent sugars, then it may empty faster from the stomach (as watermelon does), and potentially it could have a higher GI value than maple syrup's. There are other claims about its nutritional benefits, including vitamins, minerals, and polyphenols. However, we still think that it's one for the occasional category, not for everyday hydration. It's the calories that not only count, but add up faster than you think. To quench thirst, it's hard to beat water—sparkling or tap.[29]

MELEZITOSE

The triose melezitose is composed of two ▶**glucose** molecules and one ▶**fructose** molecule, which can be broken down to glucose and the ▶**disaccharide** turanose. It is produced by many plant-sap-eating insects, including aphids. As such, melezitose is part of ▶**honeydew**.

MESQUITE FLOUR OR POWDER

(mesquite bean flour, mesquite pod meal)

Mesquite generally brings to mind barbecue fuel, fine furniture, and fence posts (or, in parts of the world, an invasive weed to be eradicated). But mesquite pods can also be made into flour, a staple for North and South American Indians long before the arrival of Europeans. This flour also sustained early explorers: Pedro de Castañeda, who was part of the 1540–1542 Coronado Expedition, describes a "bread of mesquite, which like cheese keeps for a year"; and Hernando Ruiz de Alarcón, who traveled from Acapulco up the Colorado River in 1540, describes cakes of corn and mesquite.

Sweet mesquite flour (also called meal or powder) is now finding new life in ▶**organic** and whole food stores, although it does tend to be very pricey. The flour is milled from the wild-harvested pods of several varieties of mesquite trees (*Prosopis* genus), which, like their cousin the ▶**carob**, belong to the pea family. These pods are not starchy like bean pods. Their ▶**carbohydrate** content is mostly ▶**sucrose** plus small amounts of ▶**glucose** and ▶**fructose**. The pods' sugar content varies considerably, ranging from 5 percent for Mexico's *P. articulata* up to 37 to 38 percent for Argentina's *P. alba* and *P. nigra*. In addition, since the flour is milled from the fleshy portion of the pod rather than the seed, it has none of the gassy side effects of other bean flours.

The sugar content of commercial mesquite flours ranges from about 35 percent (when the entire pod is ground) to 46 to 48 percent (when only the mesocarp, or the fleshy part of the fruit, is ground) for Peru's *P. pallida* and up to 59 percent for *P. alba* from Argentina. These flours are also rich in dietary ▶**fiber** (some 28 percent) and provide similar amounts of protein, as do corn (maize), sorghum, oats, and rice. Mesquite has a low glycemic index (GI 25) and was one of the first foods tested at the University of Sydney.

This gluten-free flour has a distinctive cinnamon-mocha-coconut aroma and flavor and is best used to replace a small portion of flour in recipes for breads, muffins, cookies, cakes, pancakes, tortillas, etc. You can also add it to milky drinks and shakes for extra zing. In Peru, the pods (from *P. Pallida*) are used to make *algarrobina*, a syrup reminiscent of carob syrup.

Plant scientist Peter Felker told us that he had expected that mesquite flour's major market would be gluten-free, but, in fact, the serious demand is for desserts in general, thanks to the unique aroma and flavor synergy of mesquite flour and chocolate.

You can buy mesquite flour online and from specialty whole food and organic stores. However, even these dedicated retailers find it hard to classify—when we went shopping, we found it shelved with the protein shakes and bodybuilding products, not the flours, sweeteners, or even the carob products.

For Peter Felker, mesquite flour's introduction to the market "demonstrates that mesquite forests in many parts of the world can produce much greater wealth and hundreds of local jobs in poor rural areas by harvesting their pods in addition to providing rangeland, firewood, and charcoal."

▶ MESQUITE FLOUR OR POWDER AT A GLANCE

Nutritive

Sugars Sucrose, glucose, fructose

Sweetness relative to sucrose Much less sweet (no specific data)

Calories 20 calories (84 kilojoules) per level teaspoon

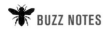 BUZZ NOTES
An Ancient Staple

Passionate plant scientist Peter Felker of Casa de Mesquite writes:

> Mesquite beans were one of the major, if not the most important, food sources of the desert Apache, Pima, Cahuilla, Maricopa, Yuma, Yavapai, Mohave, Walapi, and Hopi tribes. . . . The Indians distinguished trees that produced bitter pods from those that produced sweet, nonastringent pods, and in some tribes individual families maintained ownership of selected trees. A single grove can contain trees that vary greatly in bitterness. During the harvest season in June or July, the women and children often remained in the groves until the pod harvest was complete, after which great quantities of mesquite products were stored to provide food year-round. Many of the desert Cahuilla Indians of California stored the mesquite beans intact on the roofs of their dwellings in large elevated baskets woven of arrow weed or willow twigs and sealed with mud. The largest wicker baskets held ten to fifteen bushels each, a quantity sufficient to feed a family of six to ten people for a year. Some Maricopa Indians processed the pods prior to storage. Maricopa women pounded the pods into meal in a cottonwood or mesquite mortar, sifted the meal into fine and coarse grinds, and then poured the fine meal into an elliptical hole in the ground. The very hard seeds and the surrounding endocarp were usually discarded, as they were too difficult to grind and represented only about 10 percent of each pod. Water was sprinkled onto the meal, layer by layer, a process that hardened the ground meal with its high sugar content into a firm, dry cake. The next day the women would remove the cakes from the hole. These cakes served as the long-term-storage form of the pods. Pieces were broken off and used for daily food preparation; they also served as dry rations for men going out to hunt.[30]

MIRACULIN AND MIRACLE FRUIT

Miracle fruit (*Synsepalum dulcificum*), also known as miracle bush, miracle berry, or *asaba*, is not a sugar or a sugar substitute. It doesn't even taste sweet. But this small, bright red, bean-shaped berry causes acidic foods such as lemons and limes to taste sweet (it's apparently less effective with acidic vinegary tastes). "Chewed without being swallowed, it has the property of sweetening that which one can afterwards put in the mouth which is sour or bitter," wrote explorer Chevalier des Marchais, who, as far as we know, is the first European to have tried it, during his 1725 trip to West Africa. The taste twister in the fruit is a protein (technically a glycoprotein) that was isolated and named "miraculin" in 1968 by Japanese scientist Kenzo Kurihara. The little protein works its "miracle" by binding to the sweetness receptors on the tongue without activating them until they meet something sour or acidic; the effect lasts as long as the protein is bound to the tongue, generally up to an hour.

For some years, miracle fruit and miraculin products have been more party trick than practical. Molecular gastronomy chef Homaro Cantu, of the Chicago restaurant iNG, is renowned for his flavor-tripping dishes and cocktails that are prepared without sugar but that taste sweet after diners have dissolved a miraculin tablet over their tongue for a minute.

Potentially, miraculin has a much more serious and beneficial side, which Cantu has been involved in developing. Taste changes are very common in patients undergoing chemotherapy and can be of long duration. These changes are frequently associated with loss of appetite and poor nutrition, and they can reduce quality of life, as cancer sufferers and anyone nursing someone with cancer know only too well. A small pilot study published in *Clinical Journal of Oncology Nursing* reports that that taking a miraculin supplement did help to improve the taste of food for people undergoing chemotherapy.[31]

Fresh miracle berries are pricey, not widely available, and don't have a long shelf life. Enter miraculin pills, tablets, or granules based on freeze-dried miracle fruit pulp (plus potato or corn starch, microcrystalline cellulose, dibasic calcium phosphate, and magnesium stearate, according to the ingredients list on the package we checked out).

MISRI OR MISHRI

Misri, or *mishri*, is one of the oldest forms of sugar-crystal candy and has its origins in Persia and India, as does the word *candy* (see Buzz Notes on page 122). The large crystals are often dissolved in tea and also added with other spices and seeds to make a mouth or breath freshener. You can buy misri from Indian grocery stores and online. *See also* ▶rock sugar or candy

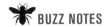
Ever Wondered Where the Word *Candy* Comes From?

Like so many of the words we use today, *candy*, it would seem, comes to us from India (from the Sanskrit *khanda*, which can mean "piece" or "fragment"). As you follow the trail to English, you journey through ancient Persia (*qand*, meaning "candied," and the Arabic *qandi*), and on to Rome (*saccharum candi)* and France (*sucre candi*), then cross the Channel with William the Conquerer in 1066, and sometime after that you discover the English *sugar candy*. It was obviously well known by Shakespeare's time, since in *Henry IV* Prince Hal finds in Falstaff's pocket "one poor pennyworth of sugar candy to make thee long-winded."

MOGROSIDES

Mogrosides are a family of cucurbitane-type triterpene glycosides that occur naturally in ▶**monk fruit**, providing its sweetness.

MOLASSES

(▶*treacle*)

Traditional recipes such as Boston baked beans, dark fruitcakes, gingerbread, spicy cookies, shoofly pie, and toffee wouldn't be the same without molasses, that thick, dark, syrupy by-product of sugar refining. It's not just for cooking. It is used in manufacturing a wide range of products from vinegars, syrups, and sauces to stouts, porters, and brown ales, as well as animal feed, fertilizers, and pharmaceuticals. It can also be fermented and distilled to produce rum, as well as ethyl alcohol. The vast majority of ethanol in India comes from ▶**sugarcane** molasses, and it is widely used in the United States and Australia as a more sustainable fuel (it is a renewable resource, unlike gasoline, which is a fossil fuel).

There's a tendency with health food fans to classify molasses as a "good" sugar because they see it as being less refined than regular white ▶**granulated sugar** and containing valuable micronutrients such as iron, calcium, and phosphorus. However, we wouldn't remove it from the "keep it moderate" category. It is still sugar, not a health food, and the quantity of its micronutrients (even in ▶**blackstrap molasses**) is best described as "trace."

The molasses you buy from the store is the concentrated syrup left over in ▶**cane-sugar**–processing after the sugar crystals are extracted. In sugar refineries, the machine that separates the molasses from the crystals is the centrifuge, essentially a special spin dryer for refining sugar. As the molasses-sugar crystal mixture (*massecuite*) spins in the perforated basket, centrifugal force pushes the liquid molasses through the holes, leaving the sugar crystals on the basket wall. Light molasses comes from the first round of centrifuging. It is the sweetest molasses and can be poured directly onto foods as a syrupy topping. Round two produces the darker and more robust molasses that adds texture, color, and aroma to baking and cooking. Blackstrap molasses, from the final spinning, has the deepest, most intense, almost bitter flavor, so you should only use it in recipes that call for it. ▶**Organic** and ▶**Fairtrade** molasses products are available.

Beet sugar molasses is produced the same way but is not a consumer product. It's used as an additive in livestock feed and in producing ethyl alcohol (ethanol), food acids, and yeasts. It is also now appearing in innovative products to de-ice roads. Apparently the ▶**carbohydrates** in molasses can prevent ice from sticking to roads and keep the salt working at temperatures as low as 25°F (-4°C).

Not all "molasses" is a by-product of sugar refining. The term has long been applied to thick, ▶**honey**-like, dark-colored syrups made from fruit and grains—hence ▶**date molasses**, ▶**grape molasses**, ▶**pomegranate molasses**, and ▶**sorghum molasses**.

▶ **MOLASSES AT A GLANCE**

Nutritive

Sugars Sucrose, fructose, glucose

Sweetness relative to sucrose About 25–50% less sweet (varies; depends on grade)

Calories 16 calories (67 kilojoules) per level teaspoon

MONATIN

Monatin is a sweet-tasting ▶**protein** that was isolated in 1988 from the root of *Sclerochiton ilicifolius*, a shrub native to South Africa's Transvaal region. The root has long been known for its sweetness—it is locally called *molomo monate*, which literally means "mouth nice." Despite its high sweetness (3,000 times sweeter than sucrose), clean taste, and no noticeable aftertaste, it currently has no commercial applications and no regulatory approval. If patent literature is anything to go by, there's plenty of interest in it for a wide range of foods and beverages, including tabletop sweeteners, dairy products, sweets, and chewing gum. According to Daniel Engber, writing in *The New York Times*, "In the early 2000s, scientists at Coca-Cola added the sweetener to bottles of Sprite, then left them on the roof over the weekend; by Monday morning, the soda had turned urine yellow and developed the smell of feces."[32]

▶ **MONATIN AT A GLANCE**
Nutritive
Sweetness relative to sucrose About 3,000 times sweeter
Calories 4 calories (17 kilojoules) per gram
FDA approval No

MONELLIN

Monellin is a sweet-tasting ▶**protein** that was isolated from the serendipity berry, a vine (*Dioscoreophyllum volkensii*, formerly *cumminsii*) native to the tropical rainforests of Africa. The protein, which was originally purified in 1972, is about 3,000 times sweeter than ▶**sucrose**. Its name comes from the Monell Chemical Senses Center in Philadelphia, where it was isolated. It currently has no commercial applications and no regulatory approval.

▶ **MONELLIN AT A GLANCE**
Nutritive
Sweetness relative to sucrose About 3,000 times sweeter
Calories 4 calories (17 kilojoules) per gram
FDA approval No

MONK FRUIT

(▶*luo han guo; see page 270 for brand names*)

Monk fruit (*Siraitia grosvenorii*) has long been appreciated in China for its sweetness and was typically dried and used in cooling drinks or teas and as a medicinal herb for coughs and sore throats. The fruit itself is a small melon from the *Cucurbitaceae* (gourd) family that also includes sprawling, tendril-gripping vines such as pumpkin, squash, and cucumber. The fruit's sweetness comes from its natural sugar content (▶**glucose** and ▶**fructose**) and its ▶**mogrosides**, ▶**high-intensity sugars** (technically classified as triterpene glucosides) made up of two to six glucose molecules. Mogroside V, the one that's most abundant in monk fruit, is 200 to 400 times sweeter than ▶**sucrose** and is the active ingredient in commercial monk fruit (luo han guo) extract sweeteners. Extracting involves crushing the fruit (fresh or dried), adding water to make an infusion, then filtering and spray drying it to make a creamy white powder consisting of mostly mogroside. It is also sold as a liquid extract. It has Generally Recognized As Safe (GRAS) status in the United States; is approved for use as a tabletop sweetener and food ingredient in Australia, New Zealand, and throughout much of Asia; and is approved as a tabletop sweetener in Canada.

Hot on ▶**stevia**'s trail, monk fruit is gaining increasing consumer acceptance. It is heat and acid stable, soluble in water, and able to be used as a stand-alone sweetener, food ingredient, or component of sweetener blends with other ▶**nutritive** or ▶**nonnutritive sweeteners** for reduced- and ▶**zero-calorie** products, including beverages, dairy products, cereals, candy, baked goods, and nutritional supplements. It is already finding a role in the chocolate-milk market, replacing some of the added sugar and thus cutting calories but retaining the sweetness that encourages children to choose milk, with its calcium and other nutritional goodies, rather than a soft drink.

When you use monk fruit as a tabletop sweetener, you aren't using it "neat." It is blended with other nutritive and nonnutritive sweeteners to reduce the level of sweetness to an equivalent of regular ▶**granulated sugar**, make sure it pours out of the packet easily, and give it sufficient bulk to use in food preparation and cooking. For example, a package of Nectresse™ Natural No Calorie Sweetener describes it as "a combination of deliciously sweet Monk Fruit Extract blended with other natural sweeteners (erythritol, sugar, and molasses) to bring you the rich, sweet taste of sugar without all the calories." The package label on Monk Fruit in the Raw explains that it includes ▶**dextrose** (from corn) to "dilute the very potent monk fruit extract, which is 300 times sweeter than sugar," and SkinnyGirl Monk Fruit liquid sweetener lists as its ingredients: "Water, Monk Fruit Extract, Malic Acid, Sodium Benzoate (Preservative), and Potassium Sorbate (Preservative)."

Despite many marketing claims that suggest otherwise, monk

fruit itself has not been glycemic index tested, but like most fruits, we would expect it is moderate or low. The pure mogrosides extracted from the fruit don't have a glycemic index because they are not carbohydrates. Tabletop sweeteners that incorporate mogrosides are mostly ▶**erythritol**, which has no effect on ▶**blood glucose** levels because most of it passes through the body undigested.

When fed to rats, mogroside V is mostly broken down by digestive enzymes and bacteria in the intestines and excreted in feces as mogrol (aglycone) and components of it. However, very small amounts of mogrol and its components are found in the blood. None of these molecules affect blood glucose levels.

When using monk fruit extract products in your baking, follow the manufacturers' instructions on substituting it for sugar. It's not possible to give any general tips, as the blends contain different bulking ingredients.

▶ MONK FRUIT AT A GLANCE

Nonnutritive
Sweetness relative to sucrose About 200–400 times sweeter
Calories 0
FDA approval GRAS status
ADI Not specified

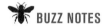

BUZZ NOTES
Plant Hunting

The "discovery" of ▶**monk fruit** was no happenstance event. It was the result of patient, persistent plant hunting by American botanists, as Walter Swingle relates in "The Source of the Chinese Lo Han Kuo," which was published in *The Journal of the Arnold Arboretum* in 1941:

> In 1932, while engaged in an agricultural survey of Kwangsi Province for the able and energetic military governor, Marshal Li Ts'ung-jen, Prof. George Weidman Groff of Lingnan University, Canton, China, discovered that the "lo han kuo," a plant widely used in household medicine in southern China, which he had been vainly seeking for many years, is cultivated in the mountains near the capital city of Kweilin by the non-Chinese Miao-tze people. Later, Prof. and Mrs. Groff visited the Kweilin region as guests of Marshal Li, who was born in this region and still maintains a residence there. On this trip visits were made to the Miao-tze villages, but no living plants

of the mysterious "lo han kuo" were seen. Marshal Li, however, sent a number of the swollen rootstocks to Prof. Groff at Canton, where they produced leafy shoots but no flowers, probably because of the high summer temperatures. These plants were the first of this species ever seen by botanists! . . .

The "lo han kuo" is a cucurbitaceous vine cultivated in northern Kwangsi by the Miao-tze people, who train it over horizontal trellises in special gardens cleared in the mountain forests. Abundant herbarium specimens and photographs of it were brought back by this expedition and turned over to me for identification. It became evident upon careful study of this material that it constitutes a new species of *Momordica* very distinct from any now known to botanists. I take pleasure in naming it *Momordica Grosvenori*, in honor of Dr. Gilbert Grosvenor, who for many years has encouraged liberally the geographic and botanical exploration of China.[33]

MONOSACCHARIDE

The simplest form of ▶**carbohydrate** is a sweet-tasting single-sugar molecule called a monosaccharide. *Mono* means one; *saccharide* means sugar. Two of the three common dietary monosaccharides come from plants:

▶**Fructose** is found in fruits, ▶**honey**, and ▶**agave** sap and has a glycemic index of 19.

▶**Galactose** is found in milk, yogurt, and whey and has a glycemic index of 15 (estimated).

▶**Glucose** is found in fruits, vegetables, grains, and honey and has a glycemic index of 100.

MUSCOVADO SUGAR

(▶*Barbados sugar, molasses sugar*)

Muscovado. This is a word that says it all. It not only describes a type of sugar, but also reminds us of the sugar industry's dark past. Christopher Columbus brought ▶**sugarcane** to the New World from the Canary Islands on his second voyage in 1493. By the eighteenth century, it had become the most prosperous crop grown in the Caribbean, which produced 90 percent of Europe's sugar supply using slave labor.

The term *muscovado* first appears in English in the sixteenth century and comes from the Portuguese *mascavado*, a variant of *mascabado*, meaning "unrefined" (of sugar). It describes the original ▶**raw sugar** produced in the sugar mills on the plantations. The sugar-cane was pressed with heavy rollers to squeeze out all the juice, which was then boiled, clarified, and poured into forms, where the liquid crystallized into first-stage sugar (muscovado) that was shipped in barrels to the refineries of Europe.

It was originally considered to be "impure" and the lowest-quality sugar. How things have changed! These days, "unrefined" (when it comes to sugars and sweeteners) suggests less processed and, thus, better for you. In fact, these sugars are partially refined, not unrefined. Creating a market for muscovado and other "cane special sugars," as manufacturers call them, such as ▶**demerara**, was a purely strategic decision. In the 1970s, refined sugars (white and brown) absolutely dominated the market. In 1977, the Mauritius Sugar Syndicate and Billington's put their heads together to develop a strategy to create product differentiation for "unrefined" (▶**non-centrifugal**) **sugars** for the emerging health food market, especially in the United Kingdom. According to Mrinal Roy, who was director of the Mauritius Sugar Syndicate at the time, "Why not use more than three-and-a-half-century-old know-how in sugar manufacture to innovatively produce from the molasses-rich cane sugar juice, natural unrefined cane special sugars and market them as finished products for consumer and industrial usage, thereby generating value-added revenue for the producers?"[34]

Mauritius, which had traditionally been a producer of bulk raw sugar exported for refining abroad, had to adopt a new production culture and invest in dedicated special ▶**cane sugar** production lines to produce the fine, soft, crystallized, sticky sugar retaining 8 to 10 percent of the ▶**molasses**. Unlike most regular ▶**brown sugars**, which are ▶**granulated sugar** with a molasses coating sprayed back on, muscovado is brown all the way through. The first boxes of Billington's light and dark muscovado sugars arrived in stores in the United Kingdom from Mauritius in 1981 and 1982 respectively. Today there are numerous brands of muscovado sold worldwide, with the Philippines emerging as a major producer, especially for Asian markets.

As with other brown sugars, the molasses content may contribute vitamins and minerals not found in regular granulated white sugar, but the amounts are way too small to count toward your recommended daily intake. It is still sugar and has the same number of calories you would get from regular sugar. So do keep your daily intake moderate, as, like all ▶**nutritive sweeteners**, it can contribute to weight gain when consumed in excessive amounts.

Muscovado (light or dark) brings its aromatic and complex flavors to spicy gingerbread, fruitcakes, coffee and chocolate cakes, brownies, fudge, and Christmas mince pies. Like soft dark brown sugar, it adds depth to chutney, marinades, and glazes and brings a delicious tang to barbecue sauce and homemade baked beans. As a specialty product, it tends to be pricey, so if need be, you can substitute light or dark brown sugar, cup for cup, in recipes that call for muscovado.

▶ MUSCOVADO SUGAR AT A GLANCE
Nutritive

Sugars Sucrose

Sweetness relative to sucrose Equally sweet

Calories 16 calories (67 kilojoules) per level teaspoon

What is the most natural sweetener?

"Natural" is one of the most popular claims for many processed foods and beverages these days. With sweeteners, especially ▶**high-intensity** ones, the "natural" label seems to be applied to anything derived from a plant (the botanical kind) no matter how distantly or how highly refined or complicated the process to isolate and extract the active ingredient. We think it is fair to say that consumers and the food industry aren't on the same page with this at all. The problem is that the term is not clearly defined and thus is wide open to interpretation.

The FDA takes a very broad view, stating that it "has not objected to the use of the term on food labels provided it is used in a manner that is truthful and not misleading and the product does not contain added color, artificial flavors or synthetic substances. Use of the term 'natural' is not permitted in a product's ingredient list, with the exception of the phrase 'natural flavorings.'"

A number of class-action cases have been filed in the United States regarding "natural" products. So far none has actually gone to trial; they have either been dismissed or settled (for example, a 2013 class-action Truvia lawsuit regarding ▶**stevia**).

For now, be wary of products with "natural" in bold type on the packaging, read ingredient labels carefully, and remember that (1) "natural" products aren't always quite what they appear to be, and (2) "natural" is not a synonym for "safe" or even good for you. It's just . . . natural.

To be truly pedantic, the only 100 percent natural sweetener is probably the one made entirely by Mother Nature: ▶**honey** from the hive.

NEOCULIN

See ▶curculin

NEOHESPERIDINE

(NHDC, neoHDC)

Neohesperidine dihydrochalcone, to give it its full name, is an ▶**artificial sweetener** derived from citrus fruit, especially bitter citrus such as Seville oranges and grapefruit. It is about 1,500 to 1,800 times sweeter than ▶**granulated sugar** (▶**sucrose**). As it can block bitter flavors, it is sometimes blended with other sugar alternatives to mask aftertastes. It is not permitted for use as a sugar substitute in the United States, but it is in Europe, Australia, and New Zealand, where you are most likely to find it used as a flavoring in baked goods, beverages, chewing gums, dairy products, sweets, and sauces and in oral-health products and pharmaceuticals.

▶ NEOHESPERIDINE AT A GLANCE

Nonnutritrive
Sweetness relative to sucrose About 1,500 to 1,800 times sweeter
Calories 0
FDA approval No
EFSA Number E959
ADI 5 mg per kilogram (2.2 pounds) of body weight (EFSA)

NEOTAME

(neohexyl aspartame)

Neotame, a derivative of the amino acids phenylalanine and aspartic acid, is about 8,000 times sweeter than ▶**granulated sugar** (▶**sucrose**). It was developed by NutraSweet and approved by the FDA in 2002 for general use across many food categories, including beverages, dairy products, frozen desserts, baked goods, and chewing gum. However, it does not appear to be widely used by the food industry, and it is not currently marketed to consumers in packet or bulk form for use as a tabletop or pourable sweetener.

It is partially absorbed in the small intestine and rapidly metabolized and excreted in urine and feces. As is the case for ▶**advantame**, although it contains phenylalanine, people with phenylketonuria

(PKU; see page 243) can use it if they wish, because such a small amount of neotame is needed to sweeten foods that exposure to phenylalanine is insignificant. As a result, the FDA does not require a label warning for people with PKU on products containing neotame.

As with ▶**aspartame**, metabolism of neotame produces small amounts of methanol, a substance naturally found in foods such as meat, milk, fruits, and vegetables.

▶ **NEOTAME AT A GLANCE**
Nonnutritive
Sweetness relative to sucrose About 8,000 times sweeter
Calories 0
FDA approval Yes
EFSA Number E961
ADI 2 mg (JECFA) per kilogram (2.2 pounds) of body weight

NON-CENTRIFUGAL SUGARS

Most sugars from ▶**sugarcane** and ▶**sugar beet** that you will find in the supermarket are ▶**centrifugal sugar** products, meaning that the crystals have been separated from the ▶**molasses** at the refinery in a machine rather like a spin dryer. Most ▶**brown sugar**, for example, is white ▶**granulated sugar** with just enough molasses sprayed back on to achieve the desired color, taste, and texture.

However, the traditional, partially processed golden to dark-brown-all-the-way-through sugars that have been produced in Asia, Latin America, and Africa for hundreds of years are still around, and there is increasing interest in niche marketing them to meet consumer demand for minimally processed sugars that retain their natural molasses content.

Including ▶**jaggery** or ▶**gur** in Asia, ▶**panela** in Latin America (▶**rapadura** in Brazil), and ▶**muscovado**, non-centrifugal sugar has long been an important part of sugarcane processing. Typically (but not only) produced by on-farm, small-scale operations, it accounts for as much as 40 percent of cane use in Colombia, the world's second largest producer, and 35 percent in India, the world's number one producer.

As "non-centrifugal" doesn't exactly trip off the tongue, manufacturers tend to describe these first-stage or partially refined sugars as "▶**evaporated cane juice**," "whole sugar," "whole cane sugar," or "unrefined" (because they haven't been additionally processed in a refinery). In this book, we tend to use "partially refined" to describe the processing; but we also refer to these sugars as "unrefined" at times, as that is what you are most likely to see on the label.

Although sometimes promoted as a "whole food," "natural," or "healthier than regular sugar," non-centrifugal sugar is still sugar. It comes with the same number of calories you will get from regular granulated sugar, and, like all ▶**nutritive sweeteners**, it may contribute to weight gain when consumed in excessive amounts. These "unrefined" sugars don't appear to have been glycemic index tested following the international method. It is possible that because of the minimal manufacturing process, which retains most of the polyphenols and other bioactive substances from the sugarcane juice, they could well have a lower glycemic index than that of regular refined ▶**sucrose** (GI 65).

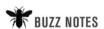
BUZZ NOTES
What's in a Name?

The best-known names for the ▶**raw**, minimally processed **sugars** produced and consumed throughout Asia, Latin America, and parts of Africa for hundreds of years are probably ▶**jaggery**, ▶**muscovado**, and ▶**panela**, but there are many more regional names. The chart below lists an international selection of names for ▶**non-centrifugal sugars**, all of which are produced in similar fashion and differ primarily in shape, size, and culinary uses.

TRADITIONAL NAME	COUNTRY
Azúcar integral, azúcar de caña integral, azúcar integral mascabo, azúcar integral mascabo	Argentina
Chancaca	Bolivia, Chile, Peru
Dulce	Costa Rica
Dulce de atado	El Salvador
Empanizao	Bolivia
Gula jawa (java), gula aren	Indonesia
Gula melaka	Malaysia
Gur	India, Pakistan, Bangladesh
Hakuru, kitul-hakuru	Sri Lanka
Jaggery	India, Pakistan, Sri Lanka, Bangladesh
Kokuto	Japan (Okinawa)

[Table continues]

TRADITIONAL NAME	COUNTRY
Mie! de panela	Venezuela
Muscovado	Mauritius, Philippines
Nam taan pep, nam taan bik, nam taan mapraou	Thailand
Pakaskas	Philippines
Panela	Colombia, Ecuador, Guatemala, Mexico, Panama, Venezuela
Panocha	Philippines
Panutsá	Philippines
Papelón	Colombia, Venezuela
Piloncillo	Mexico
Rapadou	Haiti
Rapadura	Brazil, Dominican Republic, Guatemala
Raspadura	Cuba, Ecuador, Panama
Rock sugar	China
Tapa de dulce (also dulce)	Costa Rica, Nicaragua
Vellam	Sri Lanka

NONNUTRITIVE SWEETENERS (NNS)

(▶artificial sweeteners; ▶high-intensity sweeteners; ▶zero-calorie sweeteners; see page 270 for brand names)

Nonnutritive sweeteners provide few (if any) calories (kilojoules), ▶**carbohydrates**, or any other nutrient. The category includes both ▶**artificial sweeteners** that have been created in a laboratory (e.g., ▶**aspartame**) and plant-based sweeteners whose active ingredient has been extracted from a leaf (e.g., ▶**stevia**) or a fruit (e.g., ▶**monk fruit**). Typically they are all ▶**high-intensity sweeteners**—tens, hundreds, or even thousands of times sweeter than ▶**sucrose**—so only a minute amount is needed to sweeten. Even sweeteners that do provide calories can be included under the "nonnutritive" category if they are used in such small amounts that they contribute essentially no calories to the final product. So that you can use the tabletop (pourable) versions in a similar way to ▶**granulated sugar** (e.g., by the teaspoon), the manufacturer usually adds a bulking agent such as ▶**maltodextrin** or a ▶**polyol** (sugar alcohol; e.g., ▶**erythritol**).

Nonnutritive sweeteners have virtually no effect on ▶**blood glucose** levels and can help you cut back on your calories if you use them to replace the equivalent sweetness of ▶**nutritive sweeteners** such as granulated white sugar or ▶**honey**. Their major drawback is that they aren't as versatile, because they tend not to be heat stable, they don't brown or caramelize, and they don't add texture or bulk to food when used in baking. They also tend to be much more expensive, gram for gram, than their nutritive counterparts.

A scientific statement from the American Heart Association and the American Diabetes Association concludes that "when used judiciously, NNS (nonnutritive sweeteners) could facilitate reductions in added sugars intake, thereby resulting in decreased total energy and weight loss/weight control, and promoting beneficial effects on related metabolic parameters. However, these potential benefits will not be fully realized if there is a compensatory increase in energy intake from other sources."[35]

When looking to cut calories, it's important to remember that "sugar-free" isn't code for "low-calorie." When regular sugar is replaced by nonnutritive sweeteners in energy-dense starchy or fatty foods, you may not save very many calories at all.

What about safety? Despite rigorous approval processes, controversy continues to swirl around nonnutritive sweeteners, and misinformation is massive. It is hard for the average consumer to sort fact from fiction. If you have concerns, we suggest you visit the responsible government websites such as the FDA and FSANZ, which are not only responsible for the rigorous approval process but continue to closely monitor and review new evidence about these additives on an ongoing basis.

There is strong evidence that, for most people, nonnutritive sweeteners are safe when consumed in the amounts permitted by government regulators. However, this doesn't mean that some sensitive people won't have adverse reactions to some of the nonnutritive sweeteners in foods.

Irritable bowel syndrome, which may be exacerbated by certain nonnutritive sweeteners (see **FODMAPs**), is relatively common (occurring in up to one in five people).

Food intolerance is also relatively common (up to one in five people), and people can react to a broad range of naturally occurring food chemicals such as salicylates, amines, and glutamates as well as to food additives including nonnutritive sweeteners.

If you think you may have irritable bowel syndrome or a food intolerance, look before you leap: see a registered dietitian (one who qualifies for the credential RD or RDN or, in Australia, APD) for further advice on the best alternative sweeteners.

In a 2012 paper published in the peer-reviewed journal *Diabetes Spectrum*, Claudia and her coauthors Carrie Swift and Tami Ross provide a concise summary of the FDA's review process for nonnutritive sweeteners, which must consider short- and long-term toxicity, carcinogenicity, and reproductive toxicity studies before approving these food additives. They write:

> Clinical studies examining nonnutritive sweeteners review the nutritional consequences and physiological responses of their use and determine potential toxicity levels. Toxicity is examined closely because nonnutritive sweeteners may be ingested in larger quantities than traditional additives. Studies of nonnutritive sweeteners evaluate the potential of a product or its metabolites to alter or interfere with normal absorption, metabolism, or excretion of any nutrient or metabolic intermediates, as well as any toxicological consequences. Clinical studies also consider potential allergic reactions, accumulation in tissue, levels in the stomach, effects on normal gut flora, blood glucose homeostasis, and potential drug interactions. . . . The FDA also monitors consumer complaints and conducts eating pattern surveys to determine ongoing consumption.

SWEETENER	FDA APPROVAL	TIMES SWEETER THAN SUCROSE	ADDITIONAL NOTES
Acesulfame potassium E950	Yes	200	Acesulfame potassium has no effect on blood glucose levels and doesn't provide any calories because it is not absorbed into the body.
Advantame E969	Yes	20,000	Advantame has no effect on blood glucose levels. Because it is a protein, it does provide some calories, but because it is so sweet, you only use it in minute amounts.
Alitame E956	No	2,000	Alitame has essentially no effect on blood glucose levels. Because it is a protein, it does provide some calories, but because it is so sweet, you only use it in tiny amounts.

SWEETENER	FDA APPROVAL	TIMES SWEETER THAN SUCROSE	ADDITIONAL NOTES
Aspartame E951	Yes	150–250	Aspartame has essentially no effect on blood glucose levels. Because it is a protein, it does provide some calories, but because it is very sweet, you only use it in small amounts. **WARNING**: *Aspartame should not be used by people with phenylketonuria (PKU; see page 243).*
Cyclamate E952	No	30–50	Cyclamate has essentially no effect on blood glucose levels and is not metabolized by most (75%) people.
Monk fruit/luo han guo (Mogroside V)	GRAS	200–400	Mogrosides (the active ingredient in monk fruit) have no effect on blood glucose levels and do not provide any calories, because most of them are not absorbed into the body. Not approved by the European Union.
Neotame E961	Yes	8,000	Neotame has essentially no effect on blood glucose levels. Because it is a protein, it does provide some calories, but because it is extremely sweet, it is used in absolutely minute amounts.
Saccharin E954	Yes	300–500	Saccharin has no effect on blood glucose levels and is not metabolized by the body.
Stevia (Steviol glycosides) E960	Yes	200	Steviol glycosides have zero calories and no impact on blood glucose levels because the body does not metabolize them and they are excreted.
Sucralose E955	Yes	400–600	Sucralose has no effect on blood glucose levels and does not provide any calories because it is not metabolized in the body.

[Table continues]

SWEETENER	FDA APPROVAL	TIMES SWEETER THAN SUCROSE	ADDITIONAL NOTES
Thaumatin E957	GRAS	2,000–3,000	Thaumatin has essentially no effect on blood glucose levels. Because it is a protein, it does provide some calories, but because it is so sweet, it is only used in minute amounts.

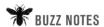 **BUZZ NOTES**

How Many Calories?

As we have explained, so that you can use the tabletop sweeteners in a similar way to ►**regular sugar** (e.g., by the teaspoon or sprinkled over your cereal), the manufacturer adds a bulking agent such as ►**malto-dextrin** or ►**erythritol**, which generally comes with a few calories. For example, each packet of Splenda® (which provides the same sweetness as two teaspoons of sugar) "has less than 1 gram of ►**carbohydrate** and less than 5 calories, which meets FDA's standards for no-calorie foods," according to the manufacturer's website.

Still, while one packet of your favorite ►**nonnutritive sweetener** may comfortably qualify for the "no-calorie" claim, if you munch on lots more products containing it over the day (or at a sitting), the calories add up, albeit slowly. So if you have a sweet tooth, it's worth checking the nutrition label of your favorite sweetener; every little bit can eventually add up to more calories than you would imagine. In the following table we have averaged out the calories from two leading brands just to give you a guide to the numbers. One packet of both Equal and Splenda is equivalent to 2 teaspoons of regular sugar (►**sucrose**).

NUMBER OF PACKETS OF EQUAL OR SPLENDA	CARBOHYDRATES (GRAMS)	CALORIES	KILOJOULES
1	1	4	17
2	2	8	34
3	3	12	50
10	10	40	160

Which nonnutritive sweeteners generate the biggest buzz within the food industry?

According to Innova Market Insights, product launches with ▶**nonnutritive sweeteners** are growing faster in the United States than products containing ▶**bulk sweeteners** (26 percent to 18 percent). Here we chart the top five nonnutritive sweeteners (as of mid-2014) and list the main products where you will find them.

SWEETENER	TOP FIVE NEW PRODUCT CATEGORIES
Acesulfame potassium	Soft drinks, confectionery, dairy, sports and energy products, desserts and ice cream
Sucralose	Soft drinks, confectionery, sports and energy products, dairy, supplements
Aspartame	Confectionery, soft drinks, dairy, snacks, fruit and vegetable products
Stevia	Soft drinks, fruit and vegetable products, sugars and sweeteners, snacks, supplements
Saccharin	Fruit and vegetable products, soft drinks, snacks, sport and energy products, sauces and seasonings

NUTRITIVE SWEETENERS

Nutritive sweeteners are those sugars and syrups that provide us with calories (energy/kilojoules). Regular white ▶**granulated sugar** is a nutritive sweetener, as are ▶**brown rice syrup** (a malted grain sweetener), ▶**sorbitol** (a ▶**polyol**, or ▶**sugar alcohol**), and ▶**maltodextrin** (a slightly sweet modified food ▶**starch**).

Regular white sugar provides calories (4.2 calories per gram, usually rounded down to 4) but little else. Other sweeteners, such as ▶**panela** or ▶**jaggery**, ▶**molasses** (▶**treacle**), wildflower (not blended) ▶**honeys**, ▶**agave nectar or syrup**, ▶**barley malt**, ▶**rice syrup**, and pure ▶**maple syrup**, provide the same number of calories plus minute amounts of minerals such as calcium, potassium, and magnesium, but not enough to contribute in any significant way to your recommended daily intake (DRI or Dietary Reference Intake).

One of the key nutritional differences among various nutritive sweeteners is their effect on your ▶**blood glucose** levels. ▶**Glucose**-rich sweeteners such as ▶**corn syrup** (GI 90) tend to have high glycemic index values, as do ▶**maltose**-rich sweeteners derived from grains, such as rice syrup (GI 98); ▶**sucrose**-rich sweeteners, such as regular ▶**brown sugar**, have moderate glycemic index values (GI 65); and ▶**fructose**-rich sweeteners, such as agave syrup (GI 19 to 28), have low glycemic index values.

The polyols (sugar alcohols), such as sorbitol, ▶**mannitol**, ▶**maltitol**, and ▶**xylitol**, are generally not as sweet as sucrose-based sugars, provide fewer calories, and have less impact on blood glucose levels. However, most have a laxative effect and may cause gas and diarrhea if consumed in large quantities. In Europe, Australia, and New Zealand, the labeling of foods containing more than 10 percent added polyols must include the advisory statement "excessive consumption may produce laxative effects." In general, they are not suitable for people with a chronic digestive problem or who need to follow a low-▶**FODMAP** diet.

Does sugar make children hyperactive?

Dietitian Nicole Senior wrote, in *GI News* in February 2010:

> The scientific jury is in—sugar is not to blame for hyperactivity in children. There is no good evidence and no plausible mechanism; however, food may still play a part—especially for a small minority of children. Sugar per se is not implicated in hyperactivity, but it is found in many foods such as confectionery and soft drinks that also contain chemicals a small number of sensitive children can react to.
>
> Hyperactivity is now known as Attention Deficit Hyperactivity Disorder (ADHD) and covers a spectrum of difficult behaviors. It has a strong genetic basis and can be affected by a variety of physiological and environmental factors, including exposure to alcohol and nicotine (from smoking) in the womb. A small number of children are sensitive to food colors and preservatives, which can result in adverse behavioral symptoms like those of ADHD. It is thought these chemicals behave more like a drug than a food on the nervous system of sensitive individuals, affecting mood, attention, concentration, and impulsivity.

Food and behavior studies are notoriously hard to construct and control because children's behavior is so easily influenced by their social setting, parenting, peer influences, and individual factors. Perhaps sugar is found in children's party foods, but they are simply responding to the excitement of a party? Maybe sugar is merely fuel for their childish energy? The myth about sugar and hyperactivity is so entrenched, there is significant bias in parents' observations too. In one study parents were asked to rate their kids behavior after a sweet drink and were told it had lots of sugar, when an artificial sweetener was secretly used instead—they all said the kids' behavior was worse. Another difficulty is, food chemical sensitivities are difficult to diagnose—there are no blood tests. It takes the skills of a specialist dietitian and an able and committed parent to complete an elimination diet and re-challenge needed to identify food chemical intolerance in a hyperactive child.

OAT SYRUP

Look for this oat-derived sweetener in the list of ingredients for products such as cereal bars, breakfast cereals, baby food, meal replacements, ice cream, yogurt, and drinks, not on the store shelf as an alternative sweetener. The products we investigated were certified ▶organic, kosher, and suitable for vegans, but the manufacturers state "presence of gluten." This is because, besides its sugars (mostly ▶maltose, plus ▶glucose and ▶sucrose), oat syrup retains some of the grain's protein during hydrolysis (the process in which the ▶starch is combined with water to break it down into its component sugar molecules), which may include gluten, especially if the oats were grown or processed alongside wheat. What about its glycemic impact? As oat syrup's main sugar is maltose, we estimate it has a high glycemic index (maltose is GI 105). As it is only slightly sweet, manufacturers need to use much more of it to get the equivalent sweetness of sucrose—and that means adding calories, too.

▶ **OAT SYRUP AT A GLANCE**
Nutritive
Sugars Maltose, glucose, sucrose
Sweetness relative to sucrose About 50% as sweet
Calories 16 calories (67 kilojoules) per level teaspoon
Health May contain gluten

OKINAWAN BLACK OR BROWN SUGAR

(▶*black sugar,* ▶*kokuto*)
▶**Sugarcane** has been grown in Okinawa since the seventeenth century. The traditional ▶**non-centrifugal** black sugar they make isn't

actually black; it is a very dark brown, unrefined sugar made by slowly cooking down the cane juice. Known locally as *kokuto*, it is a key ingredient in many traditional dishes.

OLIGOFRUCTOSE

(▶*fructooligosaccharides*)
Oligofructose belongs to a class of ▶**carbohydrates** known as ▶**fructans**, a type of soluble dietary ▶**fiber** found in plant foods such as ▶agave, artichokes, asparagus, bananas, carrots, ▶**chicory root**, garlic, Jerusalem artichokes, jicama, leeks, onions, wheat, and ▶**yacon**. You may spot it listed in ingredients labels of reduced-sugar foods and beverages, as it can be used to replace some of the sugar (▶**sucrose**, ▶**glucose**, or ▶**fructose**) in these products.

OLIGOSACCHARIDES

Oligosaccharides are chains of around three to nine single-sugar molecules (*oligo* means "a few"). They are only a little bit sweet.

▶**Fructooligosaccharides** (FOS) which are short chains of ▶**fructose** molecules, are found in plant foods such as asparagus, bananas, ▶**chicory root**, garlic, Jerusalem artichokes, leeks, onions, wheat, and ▶**yacon**.

Galactooligosaccharides (GOS) consist of short chains of ▶**galactose** molecules. They are produced through the enzymatic conversion of ▶**lactose** in milk and are prebiotics that can be only partially digested by humans. They are a preferred fuel of health-promoting bacteria in our large intestine. Mother's milk contains oligosaccharides, which remain undigested but discourage pathogens in the small intestine and facilitate the growth of friendly bacteria (e.g., *Bifidobacteria* and *Lactobacilli*) in a baby's large intestine. The beneficial bacteria produce substances that inhibit pathogenic bacteria and encourage a healthy large intestine.

▶**Maltodextrins** (modified food ▶**starches**) are chains of ▶**glucose** molecules ranging from three to nine glucose units long produced by processing a starchy food, such as corn, potatoes, rice, wheat, or tapioca, to break down the starch. They are not sugars but are commonly used as food additives to provide bulk and texture, as they are only moderately sweet or even flavorless. You will also find them in the single-serving, tabletop packet versions of some

▶**artificial sweeteners** and in pharmaceuticals. Maltodextrin is listed in the FDA's Code of Federal Regulations (CFR) as a GRAS additive, meaning it is generally recognized as safe.

Prebiotics and probiotics: A dynamic intestinal duo

Prebiotics are the non-digestible components of plant foods that help promote good gut health by stimulating the growth or activity of friendly bacteria in the large intestine. They are essentially food for the friendly (probiotic) bacteria, and they include fructooligosaccharides, such as ▶**inulin**. They are found in a broad range of plant-based foods, including artichokes, asparagus, bananas, garlic, leeks, legumes, onions, and in whole-grain foods, especially rye.

Probiotics are the friendly bacteria themselves—the live microbes that help balance our resident gut flora. You can find them in fermented foods such as yogurt, other fermented dairy foods, sauerkraut, miso, and tempeh.

ORGANIC SUGARS AND SWEETENERS

Organic is big business these days. It is also a term that can cause confusion, because different countries have different definitions of what is or isn't organic. When it comes to organic sugar and sweeteners, we suggest that you look for the "certified organic" symbol from an appropriate regulatory authority. The organic products we purchased while researching and writing this book carry various symbols representing authorities including USDA Organic, Australian Certified Organic, and NASAA Certified Organic.

The United States Department of Agriculture (USDA) has one of the world's most stringent organic certification and inspection processes. According to its website:

Organic is a labeling term that indicates that the food or other agricultural product has been produced through approved methods. These methods integrate cultural, biological, and mechanical practices that foster cycling of resources, promote ecological balance, and conserve biodiversity. Synthetic fertilizers, sewage sludge, irradiation, and genetic engineering may not be used.[36]

OUBLI

This is the fruit of *Pentadiplandra brazzeana*, a shrub or vine growing in West Africa from Nigeria east to the Central African Republic and south to Democratic Republic of Congo and Angola. Its sweetness is legendary among locals, who flavor their corn porridge with its delicious red pulp. It's called *oubli* (French for "forget") in parts of West Africa because (so the story goes) small children who eat the super-sweet berries get so distracted by them, they completely forget to go home.

▶**Brazzein** is the small sweet ▶**protein** that was originally isolated from the fruit. It is reported to be between 500 and 2,000 times sweeter than ▶**granulated sugar** (▶**sucrose**). Because of the logistical challenges of sourcing and transporting the fruit and extracting the protein, brazzein for use as a ▶**nonnutritive sweetener** is being synthesized using a special process patented by the University of Wisconsin, Madison. It has not been approved by the FDA and does not appear to be used in any foods or beverages.

PALM SUGAR

For centuries, the blossom-bearing spikes (known as inflorescence) of many palm trees—including the sugar palm (*Arenga pinnata*), the coconut palm (*Cocos nucifera*), the toddy or Asian palmyra palm (*Borassus flabellifer*), and, to a lesser extent, the date palm (*Phoenix dactylifera*)—have been tapped for their sweet sap (10 to 20 percent ▶sucrose) to produce sweet and fermented drinks, sugar, syrup, and vinegar. As palm trees are valuable, multipurpose trees in these communities, tapping the sap needs to be carried out with great skill and care to preserve the tree's well-being.

Most palm sugar (sometimes called ▶jaggery) is produced on small farms, often members of a cooperative, with varying numbers of trees. While the sap is running, to reach the inflorescence and collect the fresh sap before it begins fermenting, the farmer must climb to the top of the tree (some are up to 100 feet/30-plus meters tall) twice a day using ankle loops, aerial ropeways between trees, hoop belts, riveted bamboo, mobile and fixed ladders, and notches in the trunk. The sap is immediately boiled over open fires in a series of metal pans or woks to reduce it to a thick syrup, which is either beaten to produce granulated palm sugar or poured into coconut-shell or bamboo molds to cool, crystallize, and harden into cakes or blocks.

Like other partially refined sugars, palm sugar's ▶molasses content may contribute vitamins and minerals not found in regular ▶granulated sugar, but the amounts are far too small to count toward your recommended daily intake. Palm sugar has not been glycemic index tested following the international standard at the time of writing; however, we do know that ▶coconut sugar (which is a palm sugar from the coconut palm) has a low glycemic index (GI 54). Because of the minimal manufacturing process, which retains most of the polyphenols and other bioactive substances from the sucrose-rich sap, other varieties of palm sugar (made from the sap of sugar palms or date palms) may well have lower glycemic index values than that of regular granulated sugar (GI 65). However, if you need to manage your ▶**blood glucose** levels, we suggest you play it safe and assume that any product simply labeled "palm sugar" has a moderate glycemic index, despite manufacturers' "diabetic friendly" claims on the packaging or online.

Palm sugar is the sweetener to use in Asian cooking, especially sweets and desserts, although its caramellike sweetness also enhances curries, sauces, and dressings. Replace with soft ▶**brown sugar** if needed.

▶ **PALM SUGAR AT A GLANCE**
Nutritive
Sugars Sucrose, glucose, fructose
Sweetness relative to sucrose Equally sweet
Calories 16 calories (67 kilojoules) per level teaspoon

PANELA

(▶*chancaca, dulce,* ▶*jaggery,* ▶*rapadura*)

Panela is the most common name for the traditional sugar produced and consumed throughout Latin America and the Caribbean by concentrating freshly extracted ▶**cane juice**. Technically, it is partially refined, ▶**non-centrifugal sugar**. Although some countries (such as Brazil, Colombia, and Costa Rica) have larger-scale panela industries, most is still made in small-scale, on-farm mills (*trapiches*) with traditional technology. ▶**Sugarcane** is cut, transported to the mill (in some places still by donkey), and crushed. The freshly extracted juice is filtered, clarified, and boiled down in open pans to evaporate its water content and make a thick syrup, which is traditionally poured into molds of various shapes and sizes: cones, disks, and blocks. As the syrup cools in the mold, it crystallizes into pieces of light or dark brown compressed sugar crystals, which you grate, grind, pound (with *la piedra de la panela*, a resistant river stone), or melt to use.

Unless you are at a Latin American grocery store, the packages of panela you are most likely to find in the sugar or Latin-foods aisle of the supermarket, specialty food, or natural health store are granulated. The juice is boiled to the required concentration, and then the syrup is beaten to form free-flowing, fine, soft, golden-brown granules. It is likely to be ▶**organic** and possibly ▶**Fairtrade**, too, thus ticking the necessary boxes to satisfy growing consumer demand for less processed and more sustainably produced foods.

You may discover, as we did, claims such as "whole food," "natural," and "healthier than regular sugar" on the packaging. Remember, though, it's still sugar and comes with the same number of calories as regular ▶**granulated sugar**, so you still have to keep your daily intake moderate. As with other partially refined and/or ▶**brown sugars**, the ▶**molasses** content may contribute vitamins and minerals not found in regular sugar, but the amounts are far too small to count in any appreciable way toward your recommended daily intake. As we say elsewhere, for vitamins and minerals, the foods to choose are whole foods such as fruit, vegetables, legumes, and whole grains.

In our research, we regularly read on marketers' and producers' websites and packaging that panela has a low glycemic index, but no test data is provided. As far as we know, it hasn't been glycemic index tested following the internationally standardized method; it certainly is not on the database of glycemic index values at glycemicindex.com. It is possible that because of the minimal manufacturing process, which retains most of the polyphenols and other bioactive substances from the sugarcane juice, panela could have a lower glycemic index than regular refined ▶**sucrose** (GI 65). However, until we have the test results, we think it wise to assume the glycemic index is moderate.

Granulated panela can be used as a replacement for regular granulated sugar—brown or white—as a sweetener and in cooking. With a toffee/caramellike aroma and flavor, it is especially good for desserts and baking—cookies, cereal bars, gingerbread, muffins, carrot cakes, and fruitcakes. It also works well in sauces, marinades, and glazes and is the main ingredient in *aguapanela*, a Colombian specialty made by dissolving panela in water, to be enjoyed as is, with lemon or lime, or mixed with coffee or chocolate.

Before heading out to buy a packet of panela, you may need to familiarize yourself with its many guises. This traditional sweetener that is produced and consumed in practically all tropical and subtropical sugarcane-growing regions has numerous local names. *Panela* is probably the most common name, but Brazil's *rapadura* is the same or nearly so; ditto *dulce* from Costa Rica. It is also marketed in the United States and elsewhere as ▶**evaporated cane juice**, ▶**dehydrated cane juice**, whole sugar, and ▶**raw sugar**, to name a few. As a rule of thumb and whatever the name, if it is an organic, soft, cara-melly, golden-brown sugar from South America, it is probably panela—but you won't go wrong substituting any other partially refined non-centrifugal sugar.

▶ PANELA AT A GLANCE

Nutritive

Sugars Sucrose, glucose, fructose

Sweetness relative to sucrose Equally sweet

Calories 16 calories (67 kilojoules) per level teaspoon

Sweet records

In 2009, ninety people working twenty eight hours straight in Palmira, Colombia, made the largest and heaviest panela ever out of more than 70 tons of sugarcane. The final product measured 10 feet by 20 inches and weighed 1,576 pounds (715 kg).

PEARL SUGAR

(nib sugar; hail sugar)

Pearl sugar is a coarse, white ▶decorating sugar (▶sucrose) that provides a crunch when sprinkled on cakes and biscuits. It is tradi-tionally used on European cakes and pastries, such as German Christmas cookies, sweet Italian breads, and Swedish coffee scrolls, as it does not melt at typical baking temperatures.

PEKMEZ

(▶grape syrup)

This ▶molasses-like syrup is unfermented grape juice that has been slowly reduced over many hours to yields a concentrated sweetener that, in the days before sugar, provided an alternative source of sweetness to ▶honey in grape-growing countries. In Tur-key and the Balkans it is called *pekmez*. It's the equivalent of Italy's ▶vincotto (or **vino cotto**). It is about 10 percent sweeter than ▶granulated sugar, and its main sugars are ▶sucrose, ▶glucose, and ▶fructose, but the proportions of each vary depending on grape variety and ripeness.

PENTADIN

Pentadin is a ▶**protein** that comes from the fruit of *Pentadiplandra brazzeana*, a shrub or vine growing in West Africa from Nigeria east to the Central African Republic and south to Democratic Republic of Congo and Angola. ▶**Brazzein** also comes from this fruit. Like brazzein, it is a protein and is 500 times sweeter than ▶**sucrose.** Because it is a ▶**protein**, it provides 4 calories per gram, but because it is so sweet, it is used in very small amounts, so it will contribute virtually no calories to food. At the time of publication, it has not been commercially developed or approved for use in foods or beverages by any food authority.

▶ **PENTADIN AT A GLANCE**
Nutritive
Sweetness relative to sucrose About 500 times sweeter
Calories 4 calories per gram
FDA approval No

PILONCILLO

Piloncillo is the Mexican version of ▶**panela**. The process is the same: crushing ▶**sugarcane** to extract the juice, boiling the juice to reduce it to a concentrated syrup, pouring the syrup into the traditional cone-shaped molds that give piloncillo ("little pylon," or "little cone") its name, and allowing it to set until it is very hard. The quality of the piloncillo is indicated by its hardness since piloncillo or *panocha de piloncillo* ("pieces of piloncillo") will be grated, chopped, or ground in a *molcajete* ("mortar").
See also ▶**non-centrifugal sugar**

PLANT-DERIVED, HIGH-INTENSITY SWEETENERS

The market for plant-derived, high-intensity sweeteners, including ▶**stevia**, ▶**monk fruit**, and sweet-tasting ▶**proteins**, is growing, driven by the desire to cut costs as well as calories; food and beverage manufacturers look for ▶**alternative sweeteners** when the price of ▶**granulated sugar** (▶**sucrose**) is high.

When it comes to navigating the appropriately tough regulatory requirements and dealing with very natural consumer concerns about product safety with an alternative sweetener, "natural" credentials make life a little easier for manufacturers. "The word 'natural' is key in the development and adoption of a new generation of sweeteners by the food and beverage industry," according to Credit Suisse's *Sugar Consumption at a Crossroads* report.[37] Stevia is currently the market leader in this category, with monk fruit rising through the ranks as the only potential challenger. Of the known sweet-tasting proteins, only ▶**thaumatin** has made it to the marketplace. ▶**Brazzein** has self-affirmed GRAS status and is currently being developed as a ▶**zero-calorie sweetener** (Cweet®). At the time of publication, Cweet has not been approved for use in foods or beverages by any food authority. ▶**Curculin,** ▶**mabinlin,** ▶**monellin,** and ▶**pentadin** do not have regulatory approval in the United States or elsewhere. Nor does ▶**miraculin**, which is a taste modifier and not sweet-tasting itself.

POLYDEXTROSE

Classified by the FDA as soluble ▶**fiber**, polydextrose is technically a synthetic ▶**carbohydrate** (▶**polysaccharide** or ▶**starch**) made from ▶**glucose** (from corn), ▶**sorbitol**, and citric acid. One brand, Litesse®, describes it as a "low calorie, low glycemic (GI 4 to 7), specialty carbohydrate with prebiotic properties."

As a food additive, it provides sweetness and bulk for very few calories (because it is only partially digested), so it is used as a replacement for sugar, starch, and fat in diet and so-called "diabetic-friendly" processed foods such as candy, frozen desserts, cultured dairy products, baked goods (e.g., cakes and cookies), nutrition bars, fruit spreads, and fillings.

▶ POLYDEXTROSE AT A GLANCE
Nutritive
Sugars Glucose, sorbitol
Sweetness relative to sucrose Much less sweet
Calories 6 calories (25 kilojoules) per level teaspoon
FDA approval Yes
EFSA Number E1200
ADI Not specified

POLYOLS

(▶sugar alcohols)

Polyols, popularly known as sugar alcohols, are ▶**nutritive sweeteners**. They have been used as sugar substitutes in foods and drinks for many years, especially in "diabetic-friendly" processed products, as they provide fewer calories (an average of 2 calories or 8 kilojoules per gram, versus the 4 calories or 17 kilojoules per gram of other carbohydrates) and they have less effect on ▶**blood glucose** levels. This is because they are poorly absorbed (the body treats them like a dietary ▶**fiber**). You can find them in "sugar-free" chewing gum, candy, ice cream, baked goods, and fruit spreads. They are also used in toothpastes, mouthwashes, breath mints, and pharmaceuticals, such as cough syrups or drops and throat lozenges.

What's on the nutrition facts panel? In North America, a manufacturer will sometimes subtract the amount of polyols, along with fiber, from the total ▶**carbohydrates** per serving and add the resulting "net carbs" count to the product label as a marketing claim. Note that "net carbs" is an unregulated term in North America, and there is debate about its usefulness. In many other parts of the world including Australia and New Zealand, total carbohydrate is carbohydrate by difference (calculated by subtracting from 100, the average quantity expressed as a percentage of water, protein, fat, dietary fiber, ash, and alcohol), which is equivalent to "net carbs."

Because polyols are generally much less sweet than ▶**granulated sugar** (▶**sucrose**), food and beverage manufacturers often combine them with ▶**nonnutritive sweeteners** in foods and beverages; this will be indicated in products' ingredients lists. They are used as bulking agents to produce tabletop and spoonable or pourable forms of ▶**high-intensity sweeteners**. Apart from ▶**xylitol**, polyols on their own are not commonly used as ingredients in home cooking.

Some polyols (e.g., ▶**isomalt**, ▶**lactitol**, ▶**maltitol and maltitol syrup**, ▶**mannitol**, ▶**sorbitol**, and xylitol) may have a laxative effect and/or cause bloating, rumbling, gas, or diarrhea if you consume them in large amounts. Foods that contain more than 10 grams of lactitol, maltitol, mannitol, and xylitol per 100 grams, or more than 25 grams of ▶**erythritol**, sorbitol, or isomalt per 100 grams, carry warning statements about the possible laxative effect on their labels. These products can be a particular problem for children and adolescents because of their smaller body size. Those following a low-▶**FODMAP** diet due to digestive conditions such as irritable bowel syndrome (IBS) may especially need to avoid them. (FODMAPs are sugars in foods that are poorly absorbed by the gut. The "P" in the acronym stands for polyols.) In Europe, the labeling of foods containing more than 10 percent added polyols must include the advisory statement "excessive consumption may produce laxative effects."

The upside, however, is that they are "tooth friendly." The FDA has approved the use of a "does not promote tooth decay" health claim in labeling for sugar-free foods that contain polyols, and in other parts of the world they may be labeled "safe for teeth."

POLYOL	EXTRACTED FROM	SWEETNESS RELATIVE TO SUCROSE	FDA REGULATORY STATUS	ADDITIVE CODE NUMBER (EFSA)
Erythitol	Cornstarch	About 70% as sweet	GRAS	E968
Hydrogenated starch hydrolysate	Cornstarch	About 25–50% as sweet	GRAS	
Isomalt	Sugar (sucrose)	About 45–65% as sweet	GRAS	E953
Lactitol	Whey	About 30–40% as sweet	GRAS	E966
Maltitol	Cornstarch	About 75–90% as sweet	GRAS	E965
Mannitol	Cornstarch	About 50–70% as sweet	Approved food additive	E421
Sorbitol	Cornstarch	About 60% as sweet	GRAS	E420
Xylitol	Corncobs, birch wood waste, bagasse (cane residue after juice extracted)	Equally sweet	GRAS	E967

POLYSACCHARIDE

Polysaccharides (*poly* means "many") are not sugars; they are ▶**starches**—long chains (some branching, some straight) of single sugar molecules. Starches are not sweet at all, but they can be broken down through a series of enzymatic conversions to provide us with ▶**glucose** and ▶**maltose** sweeteners, including ▶**barley malt,** ▶**corn syrup,** ▶**oat syrup,** ▶**rice syrup,** ▶**tapioca syrup,** ▶**wheat syrup,** etc.

POMEGRANATE MOLASSES

Sweet-tart pomegranate molasses is simply concentrated pomegranate juice that has been slowly reduced to a consistency similar to that of ▶**maple syrup**. As it tends to be used sparingly—most recipes call for 1 to 2 teaspoons—you won't reap the touted nutrition and health benefits of pomegranates from using it. But you will get a lot of flavor for very few calories: a teaspoon provides only 2.5 grams of sugar and 10 calories. It hasn't been glycemic index tested, but we know that pomegranate juice has a low glycemic index (GI 53).

A dash of its tangy-to-the-tastebuds flavor adds depth and richness to traditional Middle Eastern and Mediterranean dishes, such as soups, stews, and pilafs. It is also used in marinades, dressings, dips, and toppings.

You will find it in large supermarkets, quality delis, gourmet food markets, and Middle Eastern stores, or you can buy a bottle with a click online. Online, you'll also find numerous recipes for making your own with pomegranate juice, sugar, and lemon juice, but that's not the real deal. Traditional pomegranate molasses has no added sugar at all.

▶ **POMEGRANATE MOLASSES AT A GLANCE**
 Nutritive
 Sugars Glucose, fructose
 Sweetness relative to sucrose Much less sweet
 Calories 10 calories (42 kilojoules) per level teaspoon

POWDERED SUGAR

 (▶*confectioners' sugar,* ▶*icing sugar,* ▶*fondant icing sugar,* ▶*soft icing mixture*)

This is another name for confectioners' sugar, a finely ground and sifted ▶**granulated sugar** (▶**sucrose**) with a smooth texture. It is used for whipping cream; making icings, buttercream frostings, fondant fillings, fudge, candies, and other sweets; adding the finishing decorative touch to cakes and desserts; and creating glossy glazes with a smooth, satiny texture. Powdered sugar is typically blended with 3 to 4 percent cornstarch to keep it free-flowing and prevent clumping.

► **POWDERED SUGAR AT A GLANCE**
Nutritive
Sugars Sucrose (varies; typically contains about 4–5% cornstarch)
Sweetness relative to sucrose Equally sweet
Calories 16 calories (67 kilojoules) per level teaspoon

PRESERVING SUGAR

Preserving sugar is used as an alternative to regular ►**granulated sugar** for making marmalades, jams, jellies, and preserves using fruits that are naturally high in pectin, such as citrus fruits (Seville oranges, lemons, and grapefruit). It has larger crystals that dissolve more slowly and evenly than granulated sugar, reducing the risk of burning or the need for stirring and skimming. Use ►**jam setting sugar** instead when making preserves with fruits that are low in pectin.

► **PRESERVING SUGAR AT A GLANCE**
Nutritive
Sugars Sucrose
Sweetness relative to sucrose Equally sweet
Calories 16 calories (67 kilojoules) per level teaspoon

How come sugar is a preservative?

Sugar and ►**honey** are hygroscopic. This technical term simply means that they pull moisture out of their environment and in doing so deny bacteria and fungi a nice, watery place where they can live and multiply. The bacteria die of dehydration, because the sugar actually draws water from inside them. When bees process nectar to make honey, what they are actually doing is reducing the water content to about 20 percent, so the honey in the comb is about 80 percent sugar and a very inhospitable environment for microorganisms. It's also why dense fruitcakes keep for a long time. With all that dried fruit plus added sugar, fruitcakes can be around 50 or 60 percent sugars and, properly stored, will last a long time. In the past, mariners would take them on long voyages, and families would send them to relatives who lived far away. Of course, the usual dousing with brandy also acts as a sterilizer and keeps nasty microorganisms at bay.

PRIMING SUGARS AND SYRUPS

The simplest way to carbonate beer naturally is to add a little sugar to the brew. Home brewers mostly use ▶**glucose**/▶**dextrose** (▶**corn sugar**), ▶**granulated sugar** or ▶**malt** extract, but other sugars and syrups can be used. The yeast consumes the sugar and the outcome is CO_2 and alcohol. The sugars or syrups used for this process are called priming sugars. *See also* ▶**brewing sugars and syrups**

PROTEINS, SWEET-TASTING

To date, seven sweet-tasting proteins have been extracted and isolated from the fruits, seeds, and roots of various tropical plants that scientists had noticed the locals enjoyed and used to sweeten foods. Apart from ▶**thaumatin**, you won't yet find them added to foods or drinks in most parts of the world because, for a wide range of logistical, taste, and product-performance reasons, they have not been commercialized as alternative sweeteners and do not have regulatory approval. Of course, in their homelands, the actual fruits and roots that they come from have been enjoyed for hundreds (and possibly thousands) of years.

Thaumatin has been approved as a sweetener in the European Union and in several other countries, including Australia. In the United States, it has GRAS status (Generally Recognized As Safe) for use as a flavor enhancer but not as a sweetener or sugar substitute.

As they are proteins, they provide 4 calories per gram, but because such a minute amount is required to sweeten, they are considered to be ▶**nonnutritive sweeteners**.

SWEET-TASTING PROTEIN	PLANT SOURCE	SWEETNESS RELATIVE TO SUCROSE	FDA STATUS ADDITIVE CODE NUMBER (EFSA)
Brazzein	Fruit *Pentadiplandra brazzeana*	About 500–2,000 times sweeter	GRAS
Curculin (also known as neoculin)	Fruit *Curculigo latifolia*	About 500 times sweeter	Not approved
Mabinlin	Seeds *Capparis masaikai*	About 100–400 times sweeter	Not approved

SWEET-TASTING PROTEIN	PLANT SOURCE	SWEETNESS RELATIVE TO SUCROSE	FDA STATUS ADDITIVE CODE NUMBER (EFSA)
Monatin	Root *Sclerochiton ilicifolius*	About 3,000 times sweeter	Not approved
Monellin	Berries *Dioscoreophyllum volkensii* (formerly *cumminsii*)	About 3,000 times sweeter	Not approved
Pentadin	Fruit *Pentadiplandra brazzeana*	About 500 times sweeter	Not approved
Thaumatin	Fruit (arils) *Thaumatococcus daniellii*	About 2,000–3,000 times sweeter	GRAS (flavor enhancer) E957

QUESTIONS FROM THE FRONTLINE

These days, apart from the Internet, health food/▶**organic** shops are the de facto nutritional frontline: the "go-to" place where many consumers seek information about food, diet, and what to eat. Personal trainers and fitness instructors also get their fair share of these questions, as do pharmacy staff. One of our reasons for writing this book is to provide those frontline troops (including all those passionate health and nutrition bloggers), who generally have little or no formal training in nutrition and dietetics, with a practical and reliable resource to help them answer customers' and clients' questions about sugars and sweeteners.

We visited Earth Food Store, a popular health food store (and Philippa's "local") in Sydney, and asked owners Caroline Attwooll and Jonathan Cohen and their team (including Melanie Moylan and Nick Doebeli) what questions their customers ask time and again about sugars. It became clear that many people are very confused by "label lingo"—the range of names for the same product or ingredient. Food industry marketers tend to take a little (entirely legal) poetic licence with labeling to make their brand stand out from the crowd. Portraying it as more "natural" than the competition is one way to do this; hence, the term *nectar* for syrup, or *evaporated cane juice* for sugar. Many of these topics are covered in general terms elsewhere in this book, but we thought it would be helpful to answer the questions people ask all the time in one section—"Q." Not only do you get the answers you are looking for, but also, any marketers who are reading this book can see how they are confusing us all.

What is the difference between ▶*rice syrup,* ▶*brown rice syrup, and* ▶*rice malt syrup?*

They are one and the same product: a malted grain syrup made from rice that contains the sugars ▶**maltose,** ▶**maltotriose,** and ▶**glucose.** It is about 70 percent as sweet as regular ▶**granulated sugar** (▶**sucrose**) and has a high GI value (GI 98). It has the same number of calories per teaspoon as sugar, but you may need to use more because it isn't as sweet.

Is ▶rice syrup gluten-free?

Most brands probably are gluten-free, but if you have celiac disease, check the label for the claims "gluten-free" or "does not contain gluten." Don't assume it is gluten-free because it is a rice-based product—some producers use barley enzymes in the malting process. For more information, see Gluten and Celiac Disease (page 241).

What is the difference between ▶agave syrup and agave nectar?

They are one and the same, although there will be flavor differences between brands and darker and lighter products. Whichever you choose, you are buying syrup made from the sap in the *piña* (heart) of the agave plant. The piña is cut out and crushed to extract the sap, which is then filtered and heated or treated with enzymes to convert the slightly sweet, watery sap into a very sweet syrup runnier than ▶**honey.** The amount of ▶**fructose** typically ranges from around 70 to 90 percent, giving agave nectar (syrup) a low glycemic index range (GI 19 to 28) and making it a popular sweetener with people who need to manage their ▶**blood glucose** levels. It has the same number of calories and grams of ▶**carbohydrates** per teaspoon as ▶**granulated sugar** (▶**sucrose**), but it is about 30 to 40 percent sweeter, so you use less.

I have heard that ▶coconut sugar is the healthiest sugar. Is that true?

Coconut sugar is sometimes promoted as a "whole food," "natural," and "healthier than regular sugar," but it's still sugar (▶**sucrose**) and comes with the same number of calories and grams of ▶**carbohydrates** per teaspoon as regular ▶**granulated sugar,** so you still have to keep your daily intake moderate; like all ▶**nutritive sweeteners,** it may contribute to weight gain, along with raising your ▶**blood glucose** levels, when consumed in excessive amounts. As with other ▶**brown** and/or unrefined **sugars,** the ▶**molasses** content may contribute vitamins and minerals not found in ▶**regular sugar,** but the amounts are far too small to count in any appreciable way toward your recommended daily intake. Coconut sugar does, however, have a low glycemic index value (GI 54). If you like a little sugar sprinkled on your oatmeal, it could be a better choice for you than regular ▶**white sugar**. It certainly has a lovely caramel flavor.

Does coconut flower nectar come from coconut flowers?

Coconut flower nectar is not nectar from coconut flowers; it is syrup (and it is sometimes called coconut syrup) made from the sap of the coconut palm's blossom-bearing spikes (inflorescence). The spikes are tapped (just as ▶**maple** trees are tapped) for their watery sap (around 12 percent ▶**sucrose**), which is then boiled down to evaporate the water and produce coconut syrup. For more information, see ▶**coconut sugar**.

What is the difference between syrup and nectar?

People make syrup either as part of food processing (reducing the sap from the maple tree down to ▶**maple syrup**) or in a saucepan at home boiling up sugar and water (▶**simple syrup**); nature makes nectar. The word means "food of the gods," and botanically, it is the sweet, watery liquid that plants produce in glands called nectaries, which may be inside or outside the flower. Its main ingredients are ▶**sucrose**, ▶**glucose**, and ▶**fructose**, but it can also contain amino acids and even toxins depending on the plant (e.g., New Zealand's tutu). Bees, butterflies, moths, birds, bats, Australia's sugar glider (a nocturnal, gliding possum) and some geckos are very efficient nectar collectors. People are not—although some of us as kids had fun sucking nectar out of flowers such as honeysuckle. And, some of us still do.

Why are there so many different kinds of ▶honey?

Honey's color and flavor depend on flowers—the bees' nectar source. And bees have many nectar sources, because there are many flowering plants. In the United States alone there are estimated to be around 300 different types of honey. Some are blended from mixed floral origins, and others are "single origin" honeys. In addition, processing produces a wide range of varieties such as waxy honeycomb, chunk honey, raw honey, creamed or whipped honey, crystallized honey, and the very runny honeys you can squeeze out of a plastic container.

THE ULTIMATE GUIDE TO SUGARS & SWEETENERS

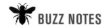 **BUZZ NOTES**

Honeypot Numbers

The 60,000 or so bees in a hive may collectively travel as much as 55,000 miles and visit more than two million flowers to gather enough nectar, drop by drop, to make one pound of honey, according to the US National Honey Board.

Which ▶honey is the healthiest?

Honey isn't a health food. It is an added sugar in the Western diet (see page 211). Although we are fans and usually have a jar in the pantry, we wouldn't remove it from the "keep it moderate" category. Some honeys do have more micronutrients and phytochemicals than others, but, even so, the amount of nutrients is best described as "trace" rather than "significant source." However, some honeys may contain added ▶**glucose** or ▶**corn syrup**, so check the label. To avoid buying "honey" that isn't 100 percent honey, but has been blended with other cheaper sweeteners, buy a local and/or certified ▶**organic** brand. And be doubly cautious if it comes in a cute-shaped container (see page 89).

How do you use honeycomb?

Comb ▶**honey** is simply honey straight from the hive just the way the bees made it, and it has been prized by our ancestors for thousands of years, as ancient rock art and engravings and paintings in caves remind us. The waxy comb is perfectly safe (if somewhat chewy) to eat, but, like honey, is not suitable for babies under twelve months. It's probably not the ideal sweetener for tea or coffee, but you can crumble it into plain yogurt or over oatmeal, pancakes, or rice pudding, and it can go places runny honey can't. For example, try topping an arugula salad with crumbled goat cheese and honeycomb. Alan was at a conference in Turkey in 2014, and honeycomb, dripping with golden sweetness, was on the breakfast buffet every morning. You had to be very quick, as it disappeared fast, he reports.

What is raw ▶honey?

There doesn't seem to be an official definition of "raw" honey, but it's generally accepted that it's honey that has not been heated (and some raw foodists would add "not filtered" to that). In the United States, the National Honey Board defines raw honey as "honey as it exists in the beehive or as obtained by extraction, settling or straining without adding heat." Raw honey fans tend to believe that it is more nutritious than honey that has been processed (i.e., heated and filtered to delay crystallization and produce a less cloudy product).

A pilot study by the National Honey Board that analyzed vitamins, minerals, and antioxidant levels in batches of raw honey that was then processed showed that while processing did significantly reduce the pollen content, it did not affect the honey's nutrient content or antioxidant activity.

In their conclusion (for those readers who want all the scientific detail) the researchers say:

> This pilot data indicates that processing honey does not result in the destruction of the key vitamins, minerals and antioxidants found in honey. In fact, processing actually increased the mineral content and AOX capacity of the honey. On average, honey's calcium, magnesium and potassium levels increased 0.8%, 14.1% and 8.9%, respectively after processing. Additionally, total antioxidant capacity increased an average of 8.4%, while hydrophilic rose 7.6% and lipophilic rose 15%. In contrast, vitamin content tended to show either no change or a slight decrease. Folic acid and Vitamin B12 experienced no measurable change during heating and filtration, and pyridoxine dropped 9.6%. As expected, pollen was completely eliminated after processing.[38]

Is ▸evaporated cane juice the same as ▸cane juice?

Evaporated cane juice is sugar described in three words rather than one. It's not your regular white ▸granulated sugar they are talking about; it is dried ▸cane syrup: South and Central America's ▸non-centrifugal sugars, such as ▸panela. ▸Sugarcane juice, on the other hand, is exactly what it says it is: juice (sap) that's been extracted from crushed ▸sugarcane.

I seem to "blow up" when I have ▸fructose. What natural sweetener can I have?

Sue Shepherd, PhD, diet fructose malabsorption guru and creator of the low-▸FODMAP recommends that people with this problem stick to sugars and sweeteners with more ▸glucose than fructose or a balanced amount of both, because glucose "piggybacks" fructose across the intestinal lining. It is foods with excess fructose that are problematic. This means ▸agave nectar/syrup is out for you, as it is rich in fructose. You will be fine with regular ▸brown or ▸white sugars

(▸sucrose), ▸maple syrup, ▸golden syrup, glucose (also known as ▸dextrose in powdered form); other ▸sucrose-based sugars, such as ▸coconut sugar or syrup, ▸panela, ▸jaggery, and ▸molasses; and with glucose or ▸maltose sweeteners such as regular ▸corn syrup (e.g., Karo or Aunt Jemima), ▸rice syrup, and ▸barley malt syrup. If you want a ▸nonnutritive sweetener such as ▸stevia or ▸monk fruit, check that it hasn't been bulked up with a ▸polyol (such as ▸xylitol, ▸sorbitol, or ▸erythritol), as people with fructose malabsorption may have trouble digesting polyols, too (they are FODMAPs). However, we suggest you discuss what's best for you with a registered dietitian.

Is ▸brown sugar healthier than white?

"It would be nice if there were a simple color rule for healthy eating. But there isn't," says our colleague, dietitian, and health writer Nicole Senior. "The brown/white rule seems to have come about to discourage overconsumption of sugar, salt, and flour. But brown sugar is on a par with white in the little-nutritional-value stakes." The take-home message: Although the ▸molasses in brown sugars may contribute vitamins and minerals not found in white, the amounts are too minute to count toward your recommended daily intake in an appreciable way. It still has all the calories that regular sugar has. Sugar is not a health food, and it never will be. But brown (and white) sugar can boost flavor or make some really healthy foods that are a little sour or tart-tasting on their own much more palatable.

Why are sugars sticky?

Sugars are a form of ▸carbohydrate. Carbohydrate molecules, as the name suggests, are made up of carbon, hydrogen, and oxygen atoms and tend to form rings with lots of hydrogen atoms around the outside. Water is made up of oxygen and hydrogen, so weak hydrogen bonds can form between molecules of carbohydrate and water. Sugar molecules bond well to water—they are hygroscopic. So, when sugars get wet, they tend to be sticky. The skin in our fingers contains water, particularly if we are sweating, so, when rubbing sugars between your fingers, you will feel stickiness.

▸Honey naturally contains a variety of sugars (▸fructose, ▸glucose, ▸sucrose, and ▸maltose) and water. The amount of water honey contains depends on a variety of factors, including temperature and the amount of water in the air (i.e., humidity), but it averages around 17 to 18 percent. So honeys are naturally sticky, as well!

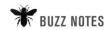 **BUZZ NOTES**

Run Rodent, Run, Run, Run!

In September 2014, a study linking ▶**artificial sweeteners** (▶**aspartame**, ▶**sucralose**, and ▶**saccharin**) to diabetes risk hit the headlines. What got lost in the hyperventilating was the fact that most of this new research was based on mouse studies. Our poor furry friends were overfed vast quantities of pure saccharin, and it altered their glucose tolerance and gut bacteria (microbiome).

Let's put this in context:

■ Saccharin has been around for over one hundred years and the "diabesity" (diabetes and obesity) epidemic has only developed over the last few decades.
■ The use of saccharin is decreasing. It is no longer a particularly popular alternative sweetener—aspartame (which was included in the study), stevia and cyclamate are much more widely used.
■ The rats were fed around 17 times more saccharin (based on the approved ADI) than a typical (Australian) adult consumes according to recent survey results.

The simple conclusion is that it's not a great idea to feed your pet mouse vast quantities of pure saccharin. "Force overfeeding rodent" studies are neither new, nor limited to artificial sweeteners. The same kinds of overfeeding experiments were carried out on rats to "prove" that fructose is toxic, for example.

The take-home? Ultimately, the dose makes the poison. Even too much water can kill you. So, the next time you see sensationalist headlines proclaiming X sweetener causes obesity/diabetes/heart disease/etc., ask the following key questions:

■ Was the research conducted in people?
■ Would you consume the amount of sweetener the subjects were fed on a regular basis over a long period of time?

If you answer no, chances are the research does not mean much to you. If you choose to use a ▶**nonnutritive sweetener** to help cut calories or manage your ▶**blood glucose levels**, do so in moderation (as in all things), and use a variety of them to reduce the likelihood of excessive consumption of any single one.

RAPADURA

This is Latin America's partially refined, ▶**non-centrifugal sugar** best known as ▶**panela**. In Brazil it is called *rapadura* and was traditionally produced as "bricks," which were grated to use in recipes or as a sweetener or cut into pieces and eaten as candy. These days, you are more likely find more convenient granulated versions of rapadura in the store, often descriptively labeled as "▶**evaporated cane juice**," "▶**dehydrated cane juice**," or "raw cane sugar."

RAW SUGAR

There are a lot of semantics involved in marketing sugars and sweeteners. If you are like most consumers, you are probably confused about what products labeled "raw," "natural," or "unrefined" really are. Are they better for us? Are they healthier in some way than regular ▶**granulated sugar**?

"Raw" certainly needs some deconstructing, because it doesn't mean "not cooked" or "in its natural state; unprocessed" as the *Oxford Dictionary* defines it. No sugar is raw in this sense. Whether made from ▶**sugarcane**, ▶**sugar beet**, or ▶**palms**, all sugar is cooked and processed (to a greater or lesser extent). It is boiled several times to remove impurities, evaporate water, and concentrate the liquid to a dark brown syrup that is then crystallized into sugar granules.

Historically, raw sugar was the minimally or partially processed commodity (▶**muscovado**) shipped from the mills on plantations in the cane-growing colonies back to the refineries in Europe. Raw sugar is still the most important internationally traded commodity, and these days very clear specifications set out the differences between raw sugar (96 to 98 percent ▶**sucrose**) and refined sugar (100 percent sucrose), because these differences determine price. It comes down to "sugar polarity," or the degree of refining purity (based on ▶**molasses** content). The four "polarity" categories are refined (white) sugar; semi-refined or direct white (also called plantation white); very-high-polarity raw sugar (VHP); and standard raw sugar.

In the store, the situation is a lot more confusing, since there are no clear definitions of "raw" sugar that consumers can rely on. You certainly can't trust the manufacturer to tell you much about the actual processing on the package or website, as that's in the realm of trade secrets and patents, although some manufacturers are much more open than others. If, for you, "raw sugar" means a less processed, specialty sugar with larger, golden-tan crystals but less moisture than a soft ▶**brown sugar,** our tip is to choose a product that has been completely processed in the country of origin, preferably ▶**Fairtrade**. Recipes that call for raw sugar typically intend the use of less refined sugars such as ▶**demerara,** ▶**Sucanat,** or ▶**turbinado sugar**.

Be aware that choosing raw sugar should be more about flavor than health benefits, because spoon for spoon, the various raw sugar products available provide the same number of calories as regular granulated sugar and probably the same moderate glycemic index (GI 65).

Although the molasses retained in raw sugar crystals may contribute vitamins and minerals not found in regular white granulated sugar, the amounts are too minute to count toward your recommended daily intake in an appreciable way. Whole foods such as fruit, vegetables, legumes, and whole grains are what you need for vitamins and minerals.

REGULAR SUGAR

(▶*granulated sugar, table sugar, white sugar*)

Regular sugar, the all-purpose pantry staple for the sugar bowl and mixing bowl, is ▶**sucrose,** a ▶**disaccharide** composed of 50 percent ▶**fructose** and 50 percent ▶**glucose**. It is refined from ▶**sugarcane** or ▶**sugar beet**. Its sweetness is the yardstick by which all other sweeteners (▶**nutritive** and ▶**nonnutritive**) are measured.

RICE SYRUP OR RICE MALT SYRUP

(▶brown rice syrup)

Although rice syrup may seem to be a relatively new-on-the-scene ingredient in health and ▶**organic** food stores, it has actually been around for a very long time. Before ▶**cane sugar** (▶**sucrose**) took center stage, rice syrup was the traditional sweetener in China and in Japan, where it is known as *mizuame* (which translates to "water candy"). It was used to make sweets and added to savory dishes to provide a glossy finish—brushed over the skin of Peking duck to achieve the magical crispy sheen, for example. Charmaine Solomon's *Encyclopedia of Asian Food* describes how in her recipe for Peking Duck, Home Style (just five ingredients): "Dissolve the ▶**maltose** (rice syrup) in hot water, brush over the duck, making sure no spot is missed. Place duck on a rack to dry in front of a window or with a fan blowing on it to speed things up a bit."

Rice syrup dissolves easily and is used in drinks and dressings, in baking, and as a topping for cereals, waffles, and pancakes. It is a popular one-for-one ▶**honey** substitute for people following a vegan diet. On the other hand, if you are substituting it for ▶**brown sugar** in a recipe, you will need to use more to achieve the equivalent level of sweetness, which also means more calories and a greater glycemic load.

This mild-flavored sweetener has an enthusiastic fan base these days, especially among people avoiding ▶**fructose**. Some fans and manufacturers claim it is "sugar-free." It is not. As a malted grain syrup made from rice, it contains the sugars maltose, ▶**maltotriose**, and ▶**glucose**. Some fans and manufacturers also say that it is a "complex, slow-digesting carbohydrate with a low glycemic index and is suitable for people with diabetes." It is not. It has a high glycemic index of 98, as you would expect with a maltose-based sweetener (maltose has a GI of 105). All of this means that it is not the ideal topping for breakfast oatmeal for people who need to manage their ▶**blood glucose** levels.

Malting has always been about alcohol as much as sweetness, so it should come as no surprise that rice syrup or rice syrup solids are used to add alcohol to and lighten the body of beers. They are used to make many American lagers and replace ▶**barley malt** in gluten-free beers. However, don't assume that rice syrup is necessarily gluten-free because it is a rice-based food product. Some producers use barley enzymes in the malting process, so check the label if you follow a gluten-free diet.

► RICE SYRUP OR RICE MALT SYRUP AT A GLANCE

Nutritive

Sugars Maltose, glucose, maltotriose

Sweetness relative to sucrose About 70% as sweet

Calories 16 calories (67 kilojoules) per level teaspoon

ROCK SUGAR OR CANDY

(►*Chinese rock sugar*)

The "rock" in this name stands for "rock hard," so if you want to keep your sweet tooth intact (and avoid a visit to the dentist), don't bite down on it. Let it dissolve. Rock sugar or candy is one of the oldest forms of sugar-crystal candy and originated in India and Persia. Arabic writers in the first half of the ninth century describe the production of candy sugar, in which crystals were grown as a result of cooling supersaturated sugar solutions (from ►**sugarcane**). The technique spread throughout the Middle East and to south and east Asia. In some parts of China, its rich and subtle sweetness makes it the sugar of choice for "red cooking" (a slow-braising cooking technique) and for sauces, marinades, sweet soups (including bird's nest and dessert soups), and sweetened chrysanthemum tea. It was also once highly regarded for its therapeutic benefits.

This is a relatively clear sugar that comes in hard yellow lumps of varying sizes that you have to crush (some people would say "whack") to get pieces small enough to measure out. To make a finer sugar, grind it down with a mortar and pestle. It is always available in Asian supermarkets. Substitute a light ►**brown sugar** if you can't find it.

► ROCK SUGAR OR CANDY AT A GLANCE

Nutritive

Sugars Sucrose

Sweetness relative to sucrose Equally sweet

Calories 16 calories (67 kilojoules) per level teaspoon; 60 calories (250 kilojoules) per "lump" (Heaven Dragon brand)

SABA

Saba is another name for the unfermented ▶**grape syrup** made in many Mediterranean countries as a sweetener and condiment that complements both sweet and savory dishes. In the store it goes by many names, depending on its country (or region) of origin. In Emilia-Romagna, Marche, and Sardinia, Italy, it is typically called *saba*. But it is also known as ▶**vincotto** (**vino cotto**) and ▶**pekmez**.

SACCHARIN

(See page 270 for brand names)

While researching coal tar, Constantin Fahlberg made the fortuitous mistake of licking his fingers and discovered the sweetener he later patented and commercialized as *saccharin* (which means "sweet like sugar"). Although soda manufacturers and canning companies quickly spotted its cost-saving potential, it didn't take off as a sugar substitute with consumers until World War I's sugar shortages. It then found an ever-expanding niche market in the calorie-counting climate of the 1960s and 1970s, when it appeared in Sweet'N Low's little pink packets alongside the sugar bowl in cafés and tearooms.

Over the years, saccharin has hurdled bumps in the regulatory road with a little help from unexpected quarters. "Anyone who says saccharin is injurious to health is an idiot," said President Theodore Roosevelt, overruling the first commissioner of the FDA, Harvey W. Wiley, in 1908. Later, in 1997, outcry from the dieting public—because there was no alternative ▶**zero-calorie sweetener** then available—pushed the US Congress into passing special legislation to put a moratorium on the FDA's proposed ban (based on a Canadian study linking it to bladder cancer in rats). However, Congress did require products containing saccharin to carry a warning label, a rule that was only repealed in 2000 after years of further research (see Q&A). Today, it is approved for use in foods and beverages in more than 100 countries worldwide.

Saccharin is a sodium salt around 300 to 500 times sweeter than regular ▶**granulated sugar** (▶**sucrose**). Because it is not metabolized by the body and is excreted in urine, it provides zero calories and has no effect on ▶**blood glucose** levels. It is often used in combination with other sweeteners in processed foods to provide "sweetness synergy," as the manufacturers put it. For example, Equal Next is a combination of saccharin and ▶**aspartame** with ▶**dextrose**. As in other ▶**high-intensity sweeteners**, bulking agents such as ▶**maltodextrin** are part of the mix in tabletop products to standardize serving sizes (so each single-serving package provides sweetness equivalent to 2 teaspoons of sugar) and create a spoonable or pourable product.

In the supermarket, you will find saccharin (or E954) listed in the ingredients of a wide range of diet foods and beverages, such as soft drinks, baked goods, jams, canned fruit, sweets, salad dressings, and toppings. It is also is used in personal care products (e.g., toothpaste, lip gloss, and mouthwash) and in pharmaceuticals and vitamins. For home use, you can choose from packets, tablets, liquids, and granulated versions.

▶ SACCHARIN AT A GLANCE

Nonnutritive
Sweetness relative to sucrose About 300–500 times sweeter
Calories 0
FDA approval Yes
EFSA Number E954
ADI 5 mg (FDA, JECFA and EFSA) per kilogram (2.2 pounds) of body weight
Health Crosses the placenta; is also secreted in breast milk

Does saccharin cause cancer?

According to the US National Cancer Institute:

> Because there is no clear evidence that saccharin causes cancer in humans, saccharin was delisted in 2000 from the U.S. National Toxicology Program's Report on Carcinogens, where it had been listed since 1981 as a substance reasonably anticipated to be a human carcinogen (a substance known to cause cancer). . . .
>
> Studies in laboratory rats during the early 1970s linked saccharin with the development of bladder cancer. For this reason, Congress mandated that further studies of saccharin be performed and required that all food containing saccharin bear the following warning label: "Use of this product may be hazardous to your health. This product contains saccharin, which has been determined to cause cancer in laboratory animals."
>
> Subsequent studies showed an increased incidence of urinary bladder cancer with high doses of saccharin, especially in male rats. However, mechanistic studies (studies that examine how a substance works in the body) have shown that these results apply only to rats. Human epidemiology studies (studies of patterns, causes, and control of diseases in groups of people) have shown no consistent evidence that saccharin is associated with bladder cancer incidence.[39]

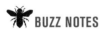 BUZZ NOTES

On July 17, 1886, *Scientific American* ran an interview with the "Inventor of Saccharine," as they put it. Here's how Dr. Constantin Fahlberg described his discovery:

> Well, it was partly by accident and partly by study. I had worked a long time upon the compound radicals and substitution products of coal tar, and had made a number of scientific discoveries, that are, so far as I know, of no commercial value. One evening I was so interested in my laboratory that I forgot about my supper until

quite late, and then rushed off for a meal without stopping to wash my hands. I sat down, broke a piece of bread, and put it to my lips. It tasted unspeakably sweet. I did not ask why it was so, probably because I thought it was some cake or sweetmeat. I rinsed my mouth with water, and dried my moustache with my napkin, when, to my surprise, the napkin tasted sweeter than the bread. Then I was puzzled. I again raised my goblet, and, as fortune would have it, applied my mouth where my fingers had touched it before. The water seemed syrup. It flashed upon me that I was the cause of the singular universal sweetness, and I accordingly tasted the end of my thumb, and found it surpassed any confectionery I had ever eaten. I saw the whole thing at a glance. I had discovered or made some coal tar substance which out-sugared sugar. I dropped my dinner, and ran back to the laboratory. There, in my excitement, I tasted the contents of every beaker and evaporating dish on the table. Luckily for me, none contained any corrosive or poisonous liquid.

One of them contained an impure solution of saccharin. On this I worked then for weeks and months till I had determined its chemical composition, its characteristics and reactions, and the best modes of making it scientifically and commercially.[40]

SANDING SUGAR AND SUGAR CRYSTALS

These large specialty crystals are specially treated to produce sparkle. They are part of a large, ever-evolving, and ever-expanding range of ▶decorating sugars that add special-occasion color and sparkle to cakes and cupcakes, cookies, and other desserts.

SIMPLE SYRUP

(bar sugar syrup; sugar syrup)

This basic mixer is an essential item at any bar for cocktail making. You can buy commercial sugar syrups or make your own: Start with one part water to one part sugar (▶confectioners' is best). Combine them in a saucepan over high heat, bring it to a boil, then reduce the heat to a simmer and stir for a couple of minutes until the sugar has completely dissolved. Set aside to let it cool to room temperature, then store in the fridge in a clean container with a well-fitting lid.

▶ SIMPLE SYRUP AT A GLANCE

Nutritive

Sugars Sucrose

Sweetness relative to sucrose Equally sweet

Calories 16 calories (67 kilojoules) per level teaspoon

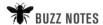 **BUZZ NOTES**

Hummers—The Feisty Feathered Kind

Hummingbirds love ▶**simple syrup**, too (in a hummingbird feeder, it's "nectar" for them). In *The Thing with Feathers: The Surprising Lives of Birds and What They Reveal About Being Human*, Noah Strycker tells the tale of a feisty hummingbird who refused to allow any other hummingbirds share the sugar syrup at the feeder. He writes:

> Liz Jones, proprietor of the Bosque del Río Tigre Sanctuary and Lodge in Costa Rica, has given up on feeding hummingbirds near her house. 'We put up our first sugar-water feeders about ten years ago,' she explained. 'It took several months for the birds to discover the feeders, but when they did, they were quite active. We had nine different species of hummingbirds making regular visits, and many of them nested in our garden. . . .
>
> Things went well with the feeder setup for a couple of years, until a feisty, rufous-tailed hummingbird arrived. Four inches long and the weight of a nickel, he was handsome enough, with an iridescent green body, red lance of a beak, and an orange-brick tail. But he was also meaner than all the other hummingbirds and never let anyone forget it. When he wasn't gorging himself on sugar, the aggressive hummer spent most of his time chasing everyone else away; this guy was the tiniest bully Liz had ever seen.
>
> She tried moving the feeder, but he just moved with it. She tried putting out more feeders so he couldn't possibly guard them all, but another roufous-tailed showed up and they joined forces to defend against all comers, in all corners of the garden. The yard rang constantly with the sound of miniature aerial dogfights.[41]

How much sugar is there in cocktails?

Not being mixologists (or even cocktail drinkers), we turned to international award-winning bartender Simon Toohey for the answer:

> Many popular cocktails, such as the mojito, include ⅔ ounce (20 milliliters) of simple (sugar) syrup, which we make ourselves with equal parts superfine (superfine/caster) sugar and water. We also use bartenders' agave syrup (not quite the same as the product in the health food store—less viscous), especially in tequila- and mesquite-based cocktails. There's a fair bit of sugar in cocktails that have fruit juice in them, too. If you want a serious I-quit-sugar cocktail without any added sugars whatsoever to save calories, you need to opt for one of the classics, such as a dry martini or a Manhattan.

Our analysis of Simon's recipes shows you save about 20 calories by opting for the sugar-free classics. But you still get a lot of empty calories, as there are 7 calories in every gram of alcohol. We put together the following chart with Simon to compare the calories from sugar and alcohol in six popular cocktails. With all the focus on sugar, people may be missing the elephant in the room—alcohol.

COCKTAIL AND INGREDIENTS	MEASURES	TOTAL CALORIES (KILOJOULES)	CALORIES FROM SUGAR	CALORIES FROM ALCOHOL
Mojito White rum Lime juice Sugar syrup Fresh mint Soda water	1-⅔ oz (50 ml) ¾ oz (25 ml) ⅔ oz (20 ml) 8 leaves 1 oz (30 ml)	150 (630 kJ)	44 (29%)	105 (68%)
Daiquiri White rum Lime juice Sugar syrup	1-⅔ oz (50 ml) ¾ oz (25 ml) 2/3 oz (20 ml)	150 (630 kJ)	44 (29%)	105 (68%)
Margarita Silver tequila Cointreau Lime juice	1-⅓ oz (40 ml) ⅔ oz (20 ml) ⅔ oz (20 ml)	155 (650 kJ)	20 (13%)	133 (84%)
Dry Martini Vodka or gin Dry vermouth	2 oz (60 ml) 1 tsp (5 ml)	130 (540 kJ)	0.4 (0.3%)	126 (98%)

COCKTAIL AND INGREDIENTS	MEASURES	TOTAL CALORIES (KILOJOULES)	CALORIES FROM SUGAR	CALORIES FROM ALCOHOL
Wet Martini Vodka or gin Dry vermouth	2 oz (60 ml) ⅔ oz (2 0 ml)	152 (640 kJ)	1.2 (1%)	147 (94%)
Manhattan American rye whiskey Sweet vermouth Angostura bitters	1-1/3 oz (40 ml) ⅔ oz (20 ml) 2 dashes	131 (550 kJ)	1.2 (1%)	126 (93%)

SORBITOL AND SORBITOL SYRUP

Sorbitol (occasionally referred to as glucitol) is a ▶**polyol** that was "discovered" in the berries of the mountain ash (*Sorbus aucuparia*) in 1872. Although it occurs naturally in many fruits and berries, today it is commercially manufactured from corn (maize), wheat, potato or cassava (tapioca). The resulting syrup may be spray dried or crystalized to obtain a powder. It is about 60 percent as sweet as regular ▶**granulated sugar** (▶**sucrose**) and, like ▶**mannitol**, has been used as a sugar substitute in a wide range of "diet" and "diabetic" processed foods for over 60 years. Today you will mostly find it in "low-sugar" or "sugar-free" chewing gum, frozen desserts, cookies, cakes, icings and fillings, toothpaste and mouthwash, and pharmaceuticals, especially chewable tablets. "The use of sorbitol far exceeds the use of all other polyols combined," according to Ronald C. Deis, PhD, director of global sweetener development for Ingredion, Inc.

It is is mainly used by the food industry as a sugar replacer or ▶**bulk sweetener** and will not be found on supermarket shelves. Crystalline sorbitol looks very much like regular sugar, but it has fewer calories, and because it is poorly absorbed (the body basically treats it as a dietary ▶**fiber**), it has virtually no effect on ▶**blood glucose** levels. Like many other polyols, sorbitol is considered "tooth friendly" but may cause bloating, rumbling, grumbling, gas, and/or diarrhea if consumed in large quantities.

► SORBITOL AND SORBITOL SYRUP AT A GLANCE
Nutritive
Sugars Sorbitol
Sweetness relative to sucrose About 60% as sweet
Calories 2.8 calories (12 kilojoules) per level teaspoon (based on US 2.6; EU 2.4; ANZ 3.3 calories per gram for labeling purposes)
FDA approval GRAS status
EFSA Number E420
ADI Not specified
LTV 23 grams per meal (JEFCA)
Health Contains ►**FODMAPs**

SORGHUM SYRUP OR MOLASSES

Sorghum is a vital cereal crop providing a staple food for millions of the world's poorest and most food-insecure people in the semi-arid tropics of Africa and Asia, and it is becoming increasingly popular in other parts of the world as a nutritious, gluten-free whole grain. There are hundreds of varieties grown for food, animal feed, syrup, alcohol, and, increasingly, ethanol, and also (possibly surprisingly) for making brooms.

The syrup comes from the sugar-rich sap of sweet sorghum (also known as Chinese sugarcane and sorgo). As with ►**sugarcane**, the stalks are crushed to extract the juice, which is then "cooked" in open pans to reduce it to the requisite thickness, along with careful skimming to remove impurities. Today, sorghum syrup is mostly an artisanal niche product, but in the latter part of the nineteenth century, it was an alternative to pricey sugar and ►**maple syrup** for many communities in the United States. It was introduced there in 1853, and cultivation was initially concentrated in the Midwest, but by the 1890s it had become a predominately Southern crop. Production reached a peak of 24 million gallons in the 1880s and then declined, because it could not compete with cheaper sugar prices and, by the twentieth century, even cheaper ►**glucose** (►**corn syrup**). US sorghum syrup production today is centered in Kentucky and Tennessee, and in bluegrass country in the Appalachians you can take part in annual celebrations such as the Morgan County Sorghum Festival.

Sorghum syrup can be used just like maple syrup and other toppings: on pancakes, waffles, toast, or ice cream; or it can be substituted, cup for cup, in any recipe that calls for ►**molasses**, ►**honey**, corn syrup, or maple syrup. It's also getting more attention as Southern chefs come to appreciate and make use of its unique flavor. "The first thing I get is this very rustic nuttiness, this umami nuttiness, then the grassiness. Then the sweetness unfolds around that," says chef Edward Lee, author of *Smoke and Pickles*. It is, according to the National Sweet Sorghum Producers & Processors Association, "that secret ingredient that gives any food that delicious taste and aroma that spells H-O-M-E-M-A-D-E."

▶ **SORGHUM SYRUP OR MOLASSES AT A GLANCE**
Nutritive

Sugars Sucrose, fructose, glucose
Sweetness relative to sucrose About 70% as sweet
Calories 20 calories (84 kilojoules) per level teaspoon

SORGHUM MALT SYRUP

This is very much a food-and-beverage industry product. Bries-Sweet™ White Sorghum Syrup is ▶**maltose** syrup made from sorghum grain as a gluten-free alternative to ▶**barley malt syrup** for brewing gluten-free beer, both commercially and for home brewers. You won't find it in the supermarket, except in ingredients lists, as the syrup can be used as a browning agent in gluten-free cereals, crackers, snack foods, and baked goods.

▶ **SORGHUM MALT SYRUP AT A GLANCE**
Nutritive

Sugars Maltose, maltotriose, glucose
Sweetness relative to sucrose About half as sweet
Calories 22 calories (92 kilojoules) per level teaspoon

STARCH

Like sugars, starches are ▶**carbohydrates** and provide 4 calories (or 17 kilojoules) per gram (so does protein). Starches are ▶**polysaccharides** (*poly* means "many")—long chains of single sugar (▶**glucose**) molecules. There are two sorts—amylose and amylopectin.

■ Amylose is a string of glucose molecule beads that tend to line up in rows and form tight, compact clumps.

- Amylopectin is a string of glucose molecules with lots of branching points, such as you see in some types of seaweed. Amylopectin molecules are larger and more open.

The starch in raw food is stored in hard, compact granules that make it difficult to digest. Most starchy foods need to be cooked for this reason. During cooking, water and heat expand the starch granules to different degrees; some granules actually burst and free the individual starch molecules. The swollen granules and free starch molecules are very easy to digest, because the starch-digesting enzymes in the small intestine have a greater surface area to attack.

Starches are not sweet-tasting at all. But they can be broken down through a series of enzymatic conversions to provide sweeteners such as ▶**barley malt**, ▶**corn syrup** and sweeteners, ▶**oat syrup**, ▶**rice syrup**, ▶**tapioca syrup**, ▶**wheat syrup**, etc. See ▶**glucose** for more details on the conversion process.

Glucose (▶**dextrose**) is available as powder, tablets, or syrup and is derived from starchy vegetables and grains including corn (maize), rice, wheat, cassava, tapioca, and potato. In the United States, cornstarch is almost exclusively used for adding bulk. Just as enzymes in our bodies break down starchy foods (such as bread, pasta, or oatmeal) into glucose molecules (see page 221), starch processors use enzymes to convert starch into a range of glucose products for the food and beverage industry. It is much cheaper and less sweet than ▶**sucrose** and has a number of practical attributes, such as adding bulk and reducing crystallization. Starch can also be fermented to produce ethyl alcohol (ethanol).

What's resistant starch?

Resistant starch is the ▶**starch** that resists digestion and absorption in the small intestine and passes through to the large intestine, where it acts like dietary ▶**fiber** to improve bowel health. Sources of resistant starch are unprocessed cereals and whole grains, firm (unripe) bananas, legumes, and starchy foods that have been cooked and then cooled, such as cold potatoes or old-fashioned oatmeal. (If you cook a pot of old-fashioned oatmeal and reheat individual portions of it each day, the heated-cooled-and-heated-again oatmeal is higher in resistant starch.) Resistant starch is also added to some refined-grain-based products, including breads and breakfast cereals, to increase their fiber content. Like other starches, it is not sweet at all.

STEVIA

(See page 270 for brand names)

Stevia's leaves contain some of the sweetest plant compounds that have been successfully commercialized as ▶**high-intensity sweeteners**. They are steviol glycosides, a type of very sweet molecule that was first commercialized in Japan in 1971. Seven glycosides have been extracted from stevia's leaves to date (stevioside, rebaudioside A, rebaudioside B, rebaudioside C, dulcoside A, rubusoside, steviolbioside). Stevioside and rebaudioside A are the two you will find in foods and beverages and in tabletop and pourable products. They have zero calories and no impact on ▶**blood glucose** levels, because the body does not metabolize them and they are excreted.

The favorite marketing word to describe steviol glycosides is "natural," because they come from a plant and are not entirely created in a laboratory beaker. Manufacturers tend to describe the extraction process as similar to making tea: steeping the leaves in water, then purifying the sweet extract. In fact, the journey through the laboratory to get to the sweetener in the packet or box is a little more complicated. Here's how it is described in the JEFCA *Compendium of Food Additive Specifications*:

> The leaves are extracted with hot water, and the aqueous extract is passed through an adsorption resin to trap and concentrate the component steviol glycosides. The resin is washed with a solvent alcohol to release the glycosides, and the product is recrystallized from methanol or aqueous ethanol. Ion-exchange resins may be used in the purification process. The final product may be spray-dried.[42]

Stevia consumer products come in sachets, tablets, liquids, and spoon-for-spoon granules. As with other high-intensity sweeteners, the ingredients list for stevia will include bulking and anticaking agents so you can pour it into a cup of coffee or measure it into your cooking and baking. In fact, when you buy stevia, you are often buying a lot of ▶**erythritol**; in some brands over 99 percent of the product is erythritol. For this reason, some products are low calorie, not zero calorie, so it is important to check the ingredients list. Before substituting stevia in your own recipes, we suggest you check out the manufacturer's website to ensure optimal results.

► STEVIA AT A GLANCE
Nonnutritive
Sweetness relative to sucrose About 200 times sweeter
Calories 0
FDA approval GRAS status
EFSA Number E960
ADI Not specified

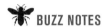 **BUZZ NOTES**

A Sweet Herb

If you want a more natural form of ►**stevia** (without ►**erythritol** or other bulking agents), dried stevia leaves and stevia leaf powder can be found in health food stores and some specialty spice shops. Here's what our colleague Ian Hemphill, spice master and author, says about stevia in his invaluable *The Spice and Herb Bible*:

> The stevia plant (*Stevia rebaudiana* Bertoni) is native to Paraguay, Brazil, and Argentina. Stevia leaves appear to have been used medicinally and as a sweet by Indians of the Guarani tribe long before Europeans came to the Americas. It was first researched by Petrus Jacobus Stevus, a 16th-century Spanish botanist the plant was originally named after. The later so-called discovery of stevia, and the identification of its use as a sweetener, has been attributed to a South American natural scientist named Dr. Moisés Santiago Bertoni, who identified it in 1887; his name now appears with the botanical name that identifies the variety used in food. In 1931, two French chemists isolated the constituent they named *stevioside* and reported it to be 200 times sweeter than sugar.
>
> Stevia . . . is a humble, spindly, soft green plant with lightly serrated wide leaves, borne in simple pairs off the soft main stem. It looks like a small weed and grows on average to less than 1½ feet (about half a meter) in height. If you want to grow it, plants are available from some herb nurseries, and it can be grown in semi-humid subtropical conditions with temperatures ranging from approximately 70°F to 100°F (20°C to 40°C). To dry the leaves, place them on screens in a dark, dry, well-aired place until they are quite crisp to the touch, indicating a moisture level of around 10%.
>
> Stevia leaf powder, which is about 30 times sweeter than sugar by volume, is deep green and has a slightly grassy aroma. The taste is intensely sweet, and the flavor has a background bitterness that

THE ULTIMATE GUIDE TO SUGARS & SWEETENERS

can be lingering if too much is eaten. To make your own stevia extract, place ½ teaspoon stevia leaf powder in ½ cup warm water. Set aside to steep overnight, then strain through a coffee filter to produce a particle-free liquid. Store the liquid in the refrigerator for up to one month.[43]

SUCANAT®

Sucanat, an abbreviation of *sucre de canne naturel* ("natural ▸**sugar-cane**") is a registered trademark. Like ▸**panela** and ▸**jaggery**, it is a partially refined ▸**cane sugar**, but it is manufactured using a proprietary drying and aeration process developed by the Swiss company Pronatec AG, founded by Albert Yersin. Eager to introduce a healthier, "tooth-friendly" sugar to Europe, Yersin and colleagues were inspired by Dr. Max-Henri Béguin's long-term studies, which showed that consuming moderate amounts of whole cane sugar as part of a healthy whole-food diet did not contribute to tooth decay (he used jaggery in his trials, apparently because he had visited India).

A Swiss pediatrician, Béguin (1918–2000) became interested in diet and cavities in the 1950s, when he noticed that tooth decay was reaching epidemic proportions among his patients. He reviewed the research of Swiss dentist Dr. Adolph Roos, who had found that in nineteenth-century Switzerland, people living in isolated mountain villages and eating wholesome, unrefined foods such as cheese, whole grains, fruits, and vegetables had good, strong teeth. Tooth decay arrived with the dietary changes that accompanied increasing accessibility to highly refined flours and sugars. Béguin came to believe that consuming refined sugar and flours, deprived of the mineral salts and vitamins contained in wholesome, natural products, was the main cause of an alarming rise in cavities.

What was Béguin's recommended whole-foods diet? It included fruits, vegetables, crudités as a side dish, whole-grain bread and whole-grain flour, milk, nuts, and unrefined (not white) sugar. He allowed 50 grams of whole cane sugar for adults a day and 40 grams for children, amounts in line with current WHO guidelines—and much less than many of us consume today.

Sucanat's fans say it is a healthier sugar. It is certainly less processed and, like other ▸**molasses**-rich sugars, it has trace amounts of minerals. But it has the same number of calories as other sugars, so it's still in the keep-consumption-moderate camp, which is what the good doctor said all along. Sucanat has not been glycemic index tested. As it contains around 93 percent ▶**sucrose** and 3 percent other sugars (▶**glucose** and ▶**fructose**), we would estimate that its glycemic index may be a little lower than regular ▶**granulated sugar** but still in the moderate range.

Sucanat can be substituted cup for cup for ▶**brown sugar**, but keep in mind that it is not crystallized and has dry, porous granules, so it will not dissolve as well as soft brown sugar.

▶ SUCANAT AT A GLANCE
Nutritive
Sugars Sucrose, glucose, fructose
Sweetness relative to sucrose Equally sweet
Calories 16 calories (67 kilojoules) per level teaspoon

SUCRALOSE

(See page 270 for brand names)

The first (and so far only) ▶**nonnutritive sweetener** made from ▶**sucrose** is sucralose. In 1976, a research team led by Queen Elizabeth College's Professor Leslie Hough, while investigating nontraditional uses of sugar for Tate & Lyle, discovered that a chlorinated sucrose derivative in the test tube was hundreds of times sweeter than sucrose (when it was accidentally tasted by chemist Shashikant Phadnis). After more than twenty years of product development and safety testing, the FDA approved Splenda as a nonnutritive sweetener in 1998 and as a general-purpose sweetener in 1999. It is now approved in more than 80 countries and is used worldwide in over 4,000 foods and drinks such as no-sugar-added fruit, diet soft drinks (including Diet Coke, Diet 7UP, and Pepsi One), and reduced-sugar juices.

Sucralose is hundreds of times sweeter than regular ▶**granulated sugar** (▶**sucrose**) and has no calories and no effect on ▶**blood glucose** levels. Radioisotope studies indicate that a small proportion (14.5 percent) is absorbed into the body and excreted mostly unchanged in the urine, while most of the rest is excreted in feces. Because it is combined with bulking agents such as ▶**maltodextrins** and ▶**dextrose** in Splenda packets, tablets, and granular products to increase the volume and make it easier to measure, these products are considered to be low-calorie sweeteners. Here are the numbers:

- One Splenda packet has 4 calories (15 kilojoules)
- One Splenda Tablet has 0.2 calories (0.8 kilojoules)
- 1 teaspoon of Splenda Granular has 2 calories (8 kilojoules)
- 1 cup Splenda Granular has 93 calories (390 kilojoules)

Splenda can be used in cooking and baking as a sugar substitute. However, as with other sugar alternatives, we suggest that, for best results, you use it in recipes already developed and tested with Splenda before substituting it for regular sugar in your family favorites.

▶ **SUCRALOSE AT A GLANCE**
Nonnutritive
Sweetness relative to sucrose About 400–600 times sweeter
Calories 0
FDA approval 1998 as a nonnutritive sweetener; 1999 as a general-purpose sweetener
EFSA Number E955
ADI 5 mg (FDA); 15 mg (JECFA & EFSA) per kilogram (2.2 pounds) of body weight

SUCROSE

Sucrose is a ▶**disaccharide** made up of two sugar molecules, one ▶**fructose** and one ▶**glucose**. It is also the scientific name for the regular white ▶**table sugar** you buy at the store. The term was coined in 1857 by English chemist William Miller from the French word for table sugar, *sucre*, and the generic chemical suffix for sugars, *-ose*. You may be more familiar with sucrose as "▶**granulated sugar**." Brown or white, it's the one in the sugar bowl.

Sucrose is the main product of photosynthesis, the process by which plants transform the sun's energy into food, so it occurs naturally in fruits and vegetables and the nectar and sap of many plants. However, ▶**sugarcane**, ▶**sugar beet**, and various ▶**palms** are the only plants that produce and store enough sucrose to make it commercially worthwhile for us to grow, harvest, and extract sugar from them.

As far as many home cooks, leading chefs, and the food industry are concerned, Mother Nature won the day with sucrose. Granulated sugar is the most common household form of sugar, with fine crystals that are easy to measure out, cream into batters, sprinkle over foods, and dissolve in drinks.

"Sweet as" is the phrase that comes to mind when talking about sucrose. The sweetness levels of all sugars and sweeteners are compared with the sweetness of sucrose, which is assigned a value of 100. The following table provides a comparison of the relative sweetness of some popular sugars and ▶high-intensity sweeteners.

SUGAR OR SWEETENER	SWEETNESS
Aspartame	150–250
Erythritol	70
Fructose	170
Glucose	70
Lactose	40
Maltitol	75–90
Maltose	30–50
Mannitol	50–70
Monk fruit	200–400
Saccharin	300–500
Sorbitol	60
Stevia	200
Sucralose	400–600
Sucrose	100
Xylitol	100

▶ SUCROSE AT A GLANCE

Nutritive

Sugars Sucrose

Sweetness relative to sucrose Equally sweet

Calories 16 calories (67 kilojoules) per level teaspoon

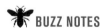 BUZZ NOTES

Sugar Can Be a Lifesaver

Diarrheal disease is a leading cause of death in children under five worldwide, responsible for killing around 760,000 children every year, particularly in poorer countries. Most of those deaths are due to severe dehydration and fluid loss. Most could be prevented by rehydration with an oral-rehydration salts solution: a mixture of clean water, salt, and sugar.

Sugar and ▶honey have long been used to help heal open wounds. For example, the people of Mesopotamia were known to wash wounds with water or milk and subsequently dress them with honey or resin. In our own times, there are well-documented cases of ▶**granulated sugar** helping to heal infected wounds and diabetic ulcers. Moses Murandu, a senior lecturer in adult nursing at the University of Wolverhampton, grew up in Zimbabwe, where his father used granulated sugar to heal wounds and reduce pain. In 2009, Murandu researched the effect of sugar on patients' wounds in the vascular ward at Selly Oak Hospital in Birmingham (United Kingdom), funding the study himself for six months. He was then awarded the prestigious Fondation Le Lous Scientific Research Innovation Award to enable him to continue his innovative work. "While salt is painful, sugar is not and reduces the pain drastically. The patients we have tested it on in the pilot study have said that they never knew such a simple method could make such a difference to their quality of life. I was happy for the patients who suffer from terrible and debilitating wounds with little hope of getting better, as this treatment can ease their pain," he said.

Sugar can be used on wounds such as bed sores, leg ulcers, and even amputations. It works because bacteria needs water to grow, and applying sugar to a wound draws the water away, thereby depriving the bacteria of water. This prevents the bacteria from multiplying, and they die. Murandu's pilot study found that a 25 percent sugar concentration ensures that the microorganisms cannot survive. Nurses were amazed by the immediate and dramatic decrease in wound odor, which enabled them to move patients from isolation to the open ward within twenty-four hours of commencing treatment, and by the marked reduction in analgesic requirements, particularly in venous-ulcer patients who had previously refused bed rest and elevation on the grounds that this position was intolerably painful.

SUGAR ALCOHOLS

"Sugar alcohols" is another name for ▶**polyols**, so-called because they are sugar alcohols that contain many hydroxyl molecules. These ▶**nutritive sweeteners** have been used as sugar substitutes in foods and drinks for many years, especially in "diabetic-friendly" processed products, as they provide fewer calories and have little effect on ▶**blood glucose** levels. They are also "tooth friendly." The downside is that some may have a laxative effect or cause gas or diarrhea if consumed in large amounts (especially for those sensitive to ▶**FODMAPs**). How do you know they are there? Well, although you won't usually see the phrase "sugar alcohol" on a label, you can spot them in the ingredients list because most sugar alcohols end in "-itol." We can't emphasize enough how important it is to read labels if you want to know what's in the processed foods you buy.

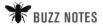

BUZZ NOTES
Sugar Bag Bees

There were not many sources of sweetness in the traditional diet of Australia's Indigenous people, but the few that existed were greatly prized and are still savored today. Reporting on the daily activities of families of nomadic Aborigines in the Northern Territory over several months in 1948, dietitian Margaret McArthur and her colleagues wrote: "An eagle eye was kept out for the stingless bee that made 'sugar bag' (yielding honeycomb about the size of the index finger). They traced the bee to the tree, where they cut out the sugar bag."

SUGAR BEET

Sugar beet (*Beta vulgaris*) is a temperate-zone crop related to root vegetables such as beets. The same *Amaranthaceae* family also includes leafy greens such as chard, spinach, and lamb's-quarters; plants grown primarily for their seeds, such as amaranth and quinoa; and a whole bunch of weeds. These cultivated crops share a common wild ancestor in the sea beet (*B. vulgaris maritima*), which grows mainly on the shore of the Mediterranean Sea and the European North Atlantic.

The history of beets as a source of sugar is a relatively short one compared with ▶**sugarcane**'s. Andreas Marggraf, a professor of physics in Berlin, was the first to extract sugar from beets in 1747. Some forty years later in 1789, Franz Karl Achard took the next step, selectively breeding beets to increase their ▶**sucrose** content and setting up the world's first beet factory in Silesia in 1801. The story then moves to France. The British blockade of the West Indies during the Napoleonic Wars meant sugar was in very short supply. Napoleon set aside one million francs to establish "sugar schools" and ordered extensive production of beets and the construction of mills to extract their sugar. By 1837, France was the largest sugar beet producer in the world. The five largest beet producers today are France, the United States, Germany, Russia, and the Ukraine, and sugar beet accounts for around 20 percent of the world's sugar supply.

Sugar beet is a biennial producing a rosette of leaves and enlarged root the first year and flowers and seeds in the second if it is left in the ground. The conical, whitish roots are about 4 inches (10 centimeters) in diameter at the top and 8 inches (20 centimeters) long and contain 20 percent sucrose when harvested.

Beet sugar is processed in one continuous procedure, without a ▶**raw sugar** stage. The sugar beets are washed, sliced, and soaked in hot water to separate the sugar-laden juice from the beet fiber. The juice is purified, filtered, concentrated, and dried in a series of steps similar to those in ▶**cane sugar** processing, resulting in ▶**granulated sugar** that is equivalent to the sucrose produced from sugarcane.

Most consumers can't tell which crop—cane or beet—the sugar in the package in their pantry came from, although experienced jam and marmalade makers and some professional bakers say they can detect a difference.

SUGARCANE

With its ▶**sucrose**-rich (16 to 18 percent) juice, sugarcane (*Saccharum officinarum*) has long been prized for its sweetness—at first simply to chew or suck on the juicy stems, later to extract the juice and boil it down to make sugar or syrup. Today, it is the source of 75 to 80 percent of the world's sugar, one of the most important internationally traded commodities. It is big business: the annual value of world sugar trade exceeds USD $24 billion, more than three-quarters of which comes from sugarcane (the balance is from ▶**sugar beet**).

This tall, perennial grass, which looks rather like bamboo, grows in tropical and semitropical regions and is propagated by cuttings. It thrives in a warm climate in rich soil with good rainfall. The stem of a mature plant can grow to 20 feet (6 meters). In many parts of the world, harvesting is still carried out by hand, and the cut and shredded canes arrive at the mill or factory within twenty-four hours, where they are crushed and boiled to evaporate off the water, leaving a dark brown syrup that is then crystallized and centrifuged to produce ▶**raw sugar** (96 to 99 percent sucrose). This is transported or exported to refineries for further processing (refining) into the various large, standard, and fine ▶**granulated sugars** and ▶**powdered sugars** that are 99.85 percent sucrose. The by-product of the refining, ▶**molasses**, is used in a wide range of products and to make rum; the cane residue, bagasse, is used as fuel, in animal feed, and in papermaking.

SUGARCANE JUICE

See ▶*cane juice*

SUGAR SYRUP

See ▶*simple syrup*

SUPERFINE SUGAR

(▶*baker's sugar,* ▶*bar sugar,* ▶*berry sugar,* ▶*caster sugar*)

▶**Granulated sugar** comes in a variety of sizes for a variety of purposes. Superfine is the finest, so it dissolves, mixes, blends, and melts very evenly. If you like to make delicate, smooth desserts such as mousse or meringues, this is the sugar to use. It can also help you create fine-crumbed baked goods, such as sponge cakes. This is because the small crystals offer more crystalline surfaces than regular granulated sugar and thus will introduce more air as you are creaming the butter (or shortening) and sugar.

▶ **SUPERFINE SUGAR AT A GLANCE**

Nutritive

Sugars Sucrose

Sweetness relative to sucrose Equally sweet

Calories 16 calories (67 kilojoules) per level teaspoon

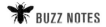 **BUZZ NOTES**

What Size Is That Sugar?

In *On Food and Cooking*, Harold McGee lays it out for us:

- Large granulated crystals—1–2 mm: coarse sugar, sanding sugar, pearl sugar
- Regular granulated sugar crystals—0.3–0.5 mm: regular table sugar (white sugar)

- Fine granulated crystals—0.1–0.3 mm: superfine sugar, ultrafine sugar, caster sugar, baker's special
- Powdered sugars—0.01–0.1 mm: confectioners' sugar, powdered sugar, icing sugar, fondant[44]

SWEET AGAVE POWDER

This is another name for ▶**agave powder**, which you should think of as a sweet dietary ▶**fiber**. It is essentially ▶**fructose** powder combined with the soluble dietary fiber (▶**inulin**) obtained from agave sap.

T

TABLE SUGAR

(▶granulated sugar, regular sugar, white sugar)

Table sugar, the all-purpose pantry staple for the sugar bowl and mixing bowl, is ▶**sucrose**, a ▶**disaccharide** composed of 50 percent ▶**fructose** and 50 percent ▶**glucose**. It is refined from ▶**sugarcane** or ▶**sugar beet**. Its sweetness is the yardstick by which all other sweeteners (▶**nutritive** and ▶**nonnutritive**) are measured.

TAGATOSE

(D-Tagatose)

Sweet-tasting tagatose is a ▶**monosaccharide** that is very similar to ▶**fructose** in its chemical structure. It is around 90 percent as sweet as regular ▶**granulated sugar** (▶**sucrose**), and it has about two-thirds the calories of sugar and virtually no effect on ▶**blood glucose** levels because it is poorly absorbed (the body basically treats it as a dietary ▶**fiber**). The same poor absorption also accounts for its very low glycemic index value (GI 3).

Tagatose is found in minute quantities in fruits, vegetables, and some dairy products (milk, yogurt, cheese) and in the gum of the tropical karaya gum tree (*Sterculia setigera*). To produce commercial quantities of tagatose, it is manufactured from ▶**lactose** from milk.

Since tagatose has received GRAS (Generally Recognized As Safe) approval from the U.S. Food and Drug Administration, it can be used in sweets, beverages, and diet products as a low-calorie sweetener. It has been also approved as a novel food ingredient in Australia, New Zealand, Brazil, Korea, Japan, and the European Union. However, it does not appear to be widely used in foods and beverages, and it is not available as a consumer tabletop product.

Like ▶**polyols** (**sugar alcohols**), tagatose has "tooth-friendly" properties. However, Food Standards Australia and New Zealand (FSANZ) came to the conclusion that foods containing tagatose may not be suitable for individuals with fructose malabsorption. So, if you need to follow a low-▶**FODMAP** diet, it may be a good idea to avoid tagatose.

▶ **TAGATOSE AT A GLANCE**
Nutritive
Sugars Tagatose
Sweetness relative to sucrose 90% as sweet
Calories 2.4 calories (2.4 kilojoules) per level teaspoon (based on US 1.5; EU 2.4; ANZ 2.6 calories per gram for labeling purposes)
FDA approval GRAS status
ADI Not specified
LTV 40 grams per meal (JEFCA)
Health Contains FODMAPs

TAPIOCA SYRUP

Finding a bottle of tapioca syrup is challenging. The only brand we were able to track down was online: Barry Farm's. Tapioca syrup is a light golden syrup that is not as sweet as ▶**regular sugar** (▶**sucrose**) but still comes with the same number of calories. It is a ▶**glucose syrup** (like ▶**corn syrup**), and, like other glucose syrups, it is made from ▶**starch**. In this case the starch comes from cassava root or yucca; the word *tapioca* itself comes from the Tupí–Guaraní *tipioca*, which refers to the starch or flour that is made by processing the roots. Being a glucose product, it is likely to have a high glycemic index (similar to corn syrup, GI 90). Cassava itself has a high glycemic index, as does boiled tapioca—GI 93, according to the database at glycemicindex.com.

Tapioca syrup is used in the food and beverage industry to add sweetness, binding, or texture to beverages, baked goods, syrups, desserts, and candies. It comes in a range of sugar profiles and varying ▶**maltose** levels, which makes it hard to be specific about its sweetness levels compared with sucrose. If you are interested in checking it out, Barry Farm suggests using it as a topping in place of ▶**maple syrup**; to add a little sweetness to smoothies; and instead of corn syrup in recipes for energy bars, muffins, and cookies.

► **TAPIOCA SYRUP AT A GLANCE**

Nutritive

Sugars Glucose, maltose

Sweetness relative to sucrose 60% as sweet (estimate; based on key sugars)

Calories 16 calories (67 kilojoules) per level teaspoon

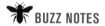 **BUZZ NOTES**

Bubble Tea

You probably know tapioca best in its "pearl" form: large or small balls of tapioca starch used in tapioca pudding or bubble tea. Bubble tea—also called boba tea, pearl tea, black pearl tea, pearl milk tea, and tapioca tea—is the "drink with the fat straw" that originated in the teahouses of Taiwan back in the 1980s and has since become a global trend. The popular name comes from the frothy bubbles on top; the alternatives "boba tea" and "pearl tea" from the starchy black tapioca pearls that sink to the bottom, providing the famous slightly gummy, chewy texture.

The original teas were black, white, or green, but fruity flavors were added early on, and today there are many variations made with fresh fruit powder, juice, pulp, or syrup that are sweetened as desired—with sugar, condensed milk, ▶**honey**, ▶**agave nectar**, or ▶**nonnutritive sweeteners**. Black tapioca pearls are the most popular addition, but many other colors are available, often matching the tea's flavor.

When you buy bubble tea from a bubble tea shop, it is typically served with an oversize straw in a clear plastic container covered with a plastic, dome-shaped lid or sealed with cellophane. The sealed cup is popular because it can be shaken and is spill-free until the cellophane is pierced. The most popular version of bubble tea is served cold, but a hot version is also available. It is easy to make at home. There are numerous recipes on the Internet and preparation demonstrations on YouTube.

THAUMATIN

(See page 270 for brand names)

Thaumatin is a ▶**high-intensity sweetener** that is about 2,000 to 3,000 times sweeter than ▶**regular** ▶**granulated sugar** (▶**sucrose**). It does provide some calories, because it is a ▶**protein**, but because it is so sweet, it is used in such minute amounts that the calories are insignificant. It has no effect on ▶**blood glucose** levels. It is currently used by the food industry more as a multifunctional flavor modifier to improve the taste profile of foods and beverages and to mask "off" tastes than as a sugar substitute, per se.

The protein is extracted from the aril of the katemfe fruit (*Thaumatococcus daniellii* Bennett) described in 1855 by Dr. William Freeman Daniell as "The Miraculous Fruit of Soudan [Sudan]" in the *Pharmaceutical Journal.* He reported considerable trade in the bright red triangular fruit and its use in local foods and drinks to "render sweet and palatable" *Aggadé* bread (a sour, corn/maize-based bread), sour fruit, and bad palm wine.

► **THAUMATIN AT A GLANCE**

Nonnutritive

Sweetness relative to sucrose About 2,000 to 3,000 times sweeter

Calories 0

FDA approval GRAS status

EFSA Number E957

ADI Not specified

 Does sugar really cause tooth decay?

Yes, and so do refined ►**maltodextrins** and ►**starches**. In fact, all highly fermentable ►**carbohydrates**—whether in the form of sugars, ►**oligosaccharides**, or starches—can contribute to tooth decay (cavities/dental caries). But, overall, sugars appear to be most likely to promote tooth decay. However, whether or not a sugary food or drink will contribute to tooth decay depends on a wide range of factors, such as how much and how often you consume the food or drink, its acidity, and its buffering power (meaning, ability to minimize the overall acidity). Constantly consuming added sugars and foods high in added sugars is clearly associated with an increased risk of developing cavities, independent of the actual amount you eat or drink. So, rather than nibble or sip them throughout the day, you are probably better off downing them in a single sitting and then brushing your teeth with fluoride toothpaste after eating. For more information on sugar and tooth decay, check out Health Matters (page 226).

TREACLE

(▶black treacle, ▶molasses)

Thick, black, and "gloopy," this classic British sugar syrup is still sold in its classic tin and exported around the world. Manufactured from the molasses by-product of the ▶**cane sugar** refining process, treacle adds color, moisture, and a rich flavor to gingerbread, Christmas pudding, parkin (a soft oatmeal cake), and treacle tart. It can also be used in glazes, barbecue sauce, and home brewing. If you want to taste the real deal, the popular Lyle's brand is available worldwide, but you can also substitute molasses, which is essentially the same thing. ▶**Golden syrup** is the lighter version.

▶ TREACLE AT A GLANCE

Nutritive

Sugars Sucrose, fructose, glucose

Sweetness relative to sucrose About 25–50% less sweet (varies; depends on grade)

Calories 16 calories (67 kilojoules) per level teaspoon

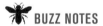 BUZZ NOTES

Take a Pound of Treakle

Traditional British gingerbread cakes were made with treacle—and lots of it! Take this example from Hannah Glasse's The Art of Cookery, Made Plain and Easy, first published in 1747. (If you're wondering, a "slack" oven is moderately warm.)

> To make Ginger-Bread Cakes. Take three Pounds of Flour, one Pound of Sugar, one Pound of Butter, rubbed in very fine, two Ounces of Ginger beat fine, a large Nutmeg grated; then take a Pound of Treakle, a quarter of a Pint of Cream, make them warm together, and make up the Bread stiff, roll it out, and make it up into thin Cakes, cut them out with a Tea-Cup, or a small Glass, or roll them round like Nuts, bake them on Tin Plates in a slack Oven.[45]

TREHALOSE

Trehalose, a ▶**disaccharide** consisting of two ▶**glucose** molecules, is the main ▶**blood glucose** in insects; you could say it's the sugar that gives bees their buzz. It was first discovered in 1832 by H. A. L. Wiggers in ergot, which is a fungal crop blight that affects rye and other cereals and has plagued civilization throughout recorded history. A quarter-century later in 1859, Marcellin Berthelot spotted trehalose again in trehala, the edible cocoons of the beetle *Larinus*, inspiring him to name the sugar "trehalose."

Trehalose is commercially produced from ▶**starch** by an enzymatic process developed by Hayashibara Co. in Japan. It is used in foods and beverages as a multipurpose ingredient—sweetener, stabilizer, thickener, and flavor enhancer. It has the same number of calories as ▶**sucrose**, so there's no particular benefit in substituting it in your cooking and baking. It is reported to be "slow digesting" because the enzyme (trehalase) that digests trehalose is found primarily in the small intestine, which means it is not fully metabolized until two or three hours after digestion. However, it has not been glycemic index tested, so we don't have the numbers to vouch for that. A small number of people have trehalase deficiency. This means they may experience gastrointestinal effects (similar to those experienced by people who are ▶**lactose** intolerant) after consuming large amounts of trehalose.

Swanson Ultra Trehalose is the only consumer product we found (available online). They say that for cooking and baking, you can replace ▶**granulated sugar** with trehalose one for one, but that because it is only about half as sweet as sugar (sucrose), you may wish to replace only a portion of the sugar in your recipe with it.

▶ TREHALOSE AT A GLANCE

Nutritive

Sugars Glucose

Sweetness relative to sucrose About 40–45% as sweet

Calories 16 calories (67 kilojoules) per level teaspoon

Health Contains trehalose

TURBINADO SUGAR

This golden-colored ▶**cane sugar** (▶**sucrose**), with large sparkling crystals and a rich aroma, is a type of ▶**raw sugar** with ▶**molasses**-rich crystals. It is similar to ▶**muscovado** and ▶**demerara**, though not identical. Mani Niall writes, in his book *Sweet!*:

> Turbinado is versatile and accommodating in all manner of cooking and baking. In butter-based doughs and batters, it creams more smoothly than demerara. But it stays crunchy when sprinkled as a topping for cookies, cobblers, and crisps. For its toffee flavor and ease of melting (its moderate-size crystals melt into larger pools than does granulated sugar), it is the best sugar for topping crème brûlée.[46]

▶ **TURBINADO SUGAR AT A GLANCE**

Nutritive

Sugars Sucrose

Sweetness relative to sucrose Equally sweet

Calories 16 calories (67 kilojoules) per level teaspoon

ULTRAFINE SUGAR

(▶baker's sugar, ▶bar sugar, ▶berry sugar, ▶caster sugar, ▶superfine sugar)

▶Granulated sugar (▶sucrose) comes in a variety of sizes for a variety of purposes. This is the finest (equivalent to superfine), so it dissolves, mixes, blends, and melts very evenly and is used for making sponge cakes and meringues.

UNREFINED SUGAR

"Unrefined," in this context, doesn't mean "not refined." All sugar, whether made from ▶sugarcane or ▶sugar beet, is partially refined (processed). It has to be boiled several times to remove impurities, evaporate water, and concentrate the liquid to a syrup that will crystallize to form the granules we call sugar. Historically, unrefined or ▶raw sugar was the partially processed commodity shipped from the mills on plantations in the cane-growing colonies back to the refineries in Europe, where it was refined.

VINCOTTO (VINO COTTO)

(▶grape syrup)

Like many Italian families in southern Italy, Angela Galtieri's made their own *vino cotto*—a condiment held in high regard and another name for grape syrup. "They only made a few liters to last them the year, as the menfolk were rather reluctant to part with their 'musto' (grape must)—they needed it for their wine," says Angela.

A few years ago, encouraged by interest from adventurous home cooks and the slow food movement, we began Il Baronello Vino Cotto (vinocotto.com.au). We had also noticed that older generations of Italians in Australia (and I imagine elsewhere in the world) no longer made their own *vino cotto* (it's very hard work) and preferred to buy it when they needed it to bake their traditional sweets such as mostaccioli (a biscuit from Calabria) and pitelli (Christmas fruit pies). They also like to use it as a dipping sauce for zeppole (Italian doughnuts), to drizzle over cartellate al vino cotto (spiral pastries), and to use in fried ravioli with chickpeas. The *vino cotto* we make is 100 percent grape syrup from late-harvest grapes that has been slowly cooked over 15 to 20 hours. It is very much an artisanal product—no large-scale production. We use an old family recipe handed down from mother to daughter over three generations. It's just grape must—no chemicals, preservatives, coloring, or red wine vinegar. We then store the syrup for a year to let the rich tones and aroma develop. We also make flavored versions— we add seasonal fruit such as figs, apples, and quince to infuse the grape syrup.

Why are some vegetables sweet?

All green plants make sugars by photosynthesis, the process by which the green chlorophyll in the plant's leaves uses sunlight (the sun's energy) to produce sugars—▶**glucose**, ▶**fructose**, and ▶**sucrose** in varying amounts and proportions. (See Buzz Notes on page 45 for more details.) Most green vegetables have only one or two grams of sugars and don't taste sweet to us at all. Here's a list of the sweeter vegetables and their (average) sugar content (raw):

   1 medium beet (beetroot) has 6 grams sugars (sucrose)

   1 medium bell pepper (capsicum) has 4 grams sugars
      (2 grams glucose + 2 grams fructose)

   1 medium carrot has 5 grams sugars (2.5 grams sucrose +
      1.4 grams glucose + 1.1 grams fructose)

   1 medium onion has 9.4 grams sugars (2.8 grams sucrose +
      4.4 grams glucose + 2.2 grams fructose)

   1 medium tomato has 3 grams sugars (1.5 grams glucose +
      1.5 grams fructose)

   1 medium ear of sweet corn has 5 grams sugars (0.3 gram
      sucrose + 2.7 grams glucose + 2 grams fructose)

   1 medium-small sweet potato has 7 grams sugars (3.4 grams
      sucrose + 2.1 grams glucose + 1.5 grams fructose)[47]

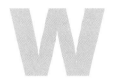

WASANBON

Wasanbon, an indispensable ingredient in *wagashi* (traditional Japanese sweets), is a specialty, handmade, fine-grained ►**granulated sugar** (►**sucrose**) made from the *chikutoh* ►**sugarcane** cultivated in Shikoku, Japan. After harvesting, the juice is pressed out of the cane and boiled down to a stage called *shiroshita-to*, meaning "sugar before it becomes white" (partially refined sugar). Here's where the refining process becomes unique. The *shiroshita-to* is allowed to stand and cool very slowly for more than a week; then the syrup is extracted and cooled again into a partially solid state. Water is added, and the sugar is kneaded by hand, placed into wooden tubs, and pressed with stones to remove more syrup. The name *wasanbon* is thought to originate from this kneading process, because it used to be done on trays (*bon*) and repeated three (*san*) times. Nowadays, kneading is repeated four or five times.

► **WASANBON AT A GLANCE**

Nutritive

Sugars Sucrose

Sweetness relative to sucrose Equally sweet

Calories 16 calories (67 kilojoules) per level teaspoon

 What is it about sugar that makes you put on weight?

Sugar has no special fattening properties. It is no more likely to be turned into fat than any other type of ►**carbohydrate**. However, sugar is often present in high-calorie foods (cakes, cookies, chocolate, and ice cream, for instance), and it's the total calories (kilojoules) in those foods, not the sugar, that's the problem. Studies have shown that diets containing a moderate amount of sugar (from a range of sources, including dairy foods and fruit) often have higher levels of micronutrients, including calcium, riboflavin, and vitamin C, than low-sugar diets.

To achieve and maintain a healthy weight, you need to keep your added-sugar intake moderate. The sugars we are talking about here are not the natural sugars in healthy foods such as fruit, but the sugars and sweeteners that we add to foods and drinks, as well as the sugars and sweeteners the food industry adds to the processed foods and drinks we buy. For more information on added sugars, see page 211.

WHEAT SYRUP

Wheat syrup is a sweetener you will find listed in the ingredients of processed foods, not on the shelves of your supermarket. It is mainly used in manufacturing sweets, beverages, jams and preserves, baked goods, cereal products, yogurts and other dairy products, condiments, and canned and packaged goods. It is derived from wheat starch in much the same way that ▶**corn syrup** is derived from cornstarch. It is composed of different sugars, mainly ▶**glucose** and ▶**fructose**, with varying compositions depending on end use. Think of it as a glucose-fructose syrup similar to ▶**high fructose corn syrup**.

Is wheat syrup gluten-free? It is such a highly processed and purified ingredient that many celiac organizations say the source of the ▶**starch** does not matter. However, if you are following a gluten-free diet, we suggest you consult your doctor or dietitian before consuming products containing wheat syrup. Better safe than sorry.

▶ WHEAT SYRUP AT A GLANCE
Nutritive
Sugars Glucose, fructose
Sweetness relative to sucrose Varies; about 70% less sweet
Calories 16 calories (67 kilojoules) per level teaspoon
Health May contain gluten

WHITE SUGAR

(▶granulated sugar, regular sugar, table sugar)

White sugar, the all-purpose pantry staple for the sugar bowl and mixing bowl, is ▶sucrose, a ▶disaccharide composed of 50 percent ▶fructose and 50 percent ▶glucose. It is refined from ▶sugarcane or ▶sugar beet. Its sweetness is the yardstick by which all other sweeteners (▶nutritive and ▶nonnutritive) are measured.

Does a spoonful of sugar cure hiccups?

Possibly. There's actually no surefire way to stop a bout of hiccups. Hiccups are usually not serious and generally last only a few minutes, but they can be annoying, as you find yourself waiting for the next one and then the next one. That's where home remedies come in, and some of them do work for some people some of the time. A spoonful of ▶granulated sugar (brown or white) is one of them. It's even been studied and written up in the prestigious *New England Journal of Medicine*, where it was reported to work in 19 out of 20 patients.[48]

Other popular possible remedies include breathing into a paper bag, drinking a glass of warm water, holding your breath, laughing loudly, eating a lemon wedge soaked in bitters, chewing on a piece of fresh ginger, and eating peanut butter. If your hiccups don't go away, see your doctor; medical treatment is occasionally necessary in chronic cases.

WOOD SUGAR

(▶birch sugar, ▶xylitol)

Wood sugar is the ▶polyol (▶sugar alcohol) xylitol, which was first used as a sweetener (isolated from birch bark) in Finland during World War II. It occurs naturally in the fibers of many fruits and vegetables but is extracted commercially from hardwoods and corncobs.

XYLITOL

(▶birch sugar, ▶wood sugar)

Discovered in 1890 by German chemist and Nobel laureate Emil Fischer, xylitol is a ▶**polyol** (▶**sugar alcohol**) that was first used commercially as a sweetener (isolated from birch bark) in Finland during World War II. It occurs naturally in the fibers of many fruits and vegetables but is extracted today from hardwoods and corncobs. Our bodies make xylitol, too—an average-size adult manufactures 5 to 15 grams of xylitol daily during normal metabolism.

Xylitol is as sweet as ▶**granulated sugar** but has fewer calories and no effect on ▶**blood glucose** levels. Like other polyols, it's "tooth-friendly," and chewing gum containing xylitol has also been shown to reduce the incidence of cavities by stimulating saliva flow—although you would have to do a lot of chewing. The downside, as with many other polyols, is its laxative effect if consumed in large quantities.

It is currently approved for use in foods, pharmaceuticals, and oral health products in more than thirty five countries. You can find it in chewing gum, gum drops, hard candy, pharmaceuticals, throat lozenges, cough syrups, children's chewable multivitamins, toothpastes, and mouthwashes.

For use in the home, xylitol, which looks like ▶**granulated sugar**, can be used spoon for spoon as a ▶**sucrose** substitute in tea and coffee, on breakfast cereal, or in your favorite recipes. We suggest that you check recipes on the manufacturers' websites before substituting it for sugar in your family favorites.

▶ XYLITOL AT A GLANCE

Nutritive

Sugars Xylitol

Sweetness relative to sucrose Equally sweet

Calories 2.4 calories (10 kilojoules) per level teaspoon (based on US & EU 2.4; ANZ 3.3 calories per gram for labeling purposes)

FDA approval GRAS status

EFSA Number E967

ADI Not specified

LTV 20 grams per meal (JEFCA)

Health Contains ▶**FODMAPs**

YACON SYRUP

Yacon (*Smallanthus sonchifolia*) is an herbaceous perennial native to the Andes, where it has been cultivated and consumed since pre-Inca times. Unlike other Andean staples, such as the potato and sweet potato, it has remained until recently a subsistence crop, with any surplus sold in nearby rural markets. The recent explosion in demand for yacon in urban centers has been mainly brought about by its popularization as a health food (AKA "superfood") with benefits for "dieters and diabetics" (a marketing promise). However, yacon syrup has not been glycemic index tested, and the original processors tend to be more cautious about making specific claims regarding its calories and glycemic impact. Most of the health claims for yacon syrup seem to be based on what we know about the health benefits of ▶**fructooligosaccharides**, which are abundant in yacon.

To make the syrup, the juice is extracted from yacon's large tuberous roots (which look rather like sweet potatoes but are sweeter and crunchier), then filtered, evaporated, and concentrated to produce a sweet syrup with a dark color and a consistency similar to that of ▶**molasses**. To obtain 2.2 pounds (1 kilogram) of syrup requires 22 to 33 pounds (10 to 15 kilograms) of washed yacon roots.

The calorie content of the syrup can vary depending on the variety of yacon used and the amount of fructooligosaccharides in the final product. These are not actually sweeteners but a type of soluble dietary ▶**fiber**, which is good for digestive health, as they have a prebiotic effect.

Live Superfoods describes its dark amber yacon syrup as having a "sweet flavour, a cross between caramel and molasses. Use it as you would honey or maple syrup on foods or in recipes or sweeten beverages with a spoonful." The Loving Earth Organic Yacon Syrup label also suggests taking a tablespoon every morning on an empty stomach to keep you regular. However, this was the most expensive sweetener we bought for our taste tests, so we suggest you use it judiciously.

▶ YACON SYRUP AT A GLANCE

Nutritive

Sugars Fructose, glucose, sucrose (also contains fructooligosaccharides)

Sweetness relative to sucrose About 50–75% as sweet

Calories 17 calories (72 kilojoules) per level teaspoon (Loving Earth brand)

Health Contains ▶FODMAPs

Z

ZERO-CALORIE SWEETENERS

(▶artificial sweeteners; ▶high-intensity sweeteners;
▶nonnutritive sweeteners; see page 270 for brand names)

Zero-calorie sweeteners provide few calories (kilojoules), ▶**carbohydrates**, or any other nutrient. The category includes artificial sweeteners, such as ▶**aspartame,** that have been created in a laboratory, as well as plant-based sweeteners, in which the active ingredient has been extracted from a leaf (e.g., ▶**stevia**) or a fruit (▶**monk fruit**). Typically they are all ▶**high-intensity sweeteners**, tens, hundreds, or even thousands of times sweeter than ▶**sucrose**, so only a minute amount is needed to sweeten. However, so you can use the tabletop (pourable) versions in a similar way to ▶**white sugar** (e.g., by the teaspoon), manufacturers usually add a bulking agent such as ▶**maltodextrin** or a ▶**sugar alcohol/polyol** (e.g., ▶**erythritol**).

Zero-calorie sweeteners have virtually no effect on ▶**blood glucose** levels and can help you cut back on your calories if you use them to replace the equivalent sweetness of ▶**granulated sugar**, ▶**honey**, etc. Their major drawback is that they aren't as versatile as ▶**nutritive sweeteners**, because they tend not to be heat stable, don't brown or caramelize, and don't add texture or bulk to food when used in baking. They also tend to be much more expensive, gram for gram, than their nutritive counterparts.

PART

2

HEALTH
MATTERS

ADDED SUGARS EQUAL ADDED CALORIES

Many delicious and nutrient-rich foods such as fruits and berries, milk, and yogurt contain sugars such as ▶**glucose**, ▶**fructose**, ▶**sucrose**, and ▶**lactose** naturally. These natural sugars provide energy for our bodies and are not a problem; most of us need to eat more fruit, not less. Dairy foods are also a great source of protein, calcium, and vitamin D, and most of us do not eat the recommended number of servings each day.

With so many people struggling to achieve and maintain a healthy weight, it's added sugars that add extra calories that are the concern. Added sugars are the sugars and ▶**nutritive sweeteners** we add to our foods and drinks (a splash of ▶**maple syrup** on a buckwheat pancake, a couple of teaspoons of ▶**honey** in a cup of tea, or the ▶**granulated sugar** used in a batch of brownies), as well as those that the food industry adds to the processed foods and drinks we buy.

According to a study published in 2014 in the peer-reviewed journal *JAMA Internal Medicine*, Americans typically consumed nearly 15 percent (300 calories) of their daily calories (2,000 calories) from added sugar between the years 2005 to 2010 (the most recent period for which there is data).[49] The major sources of these added sugars and calories in that period were sugar-sweetened beverages, grain-based desserts, fruit drinks, dairy desserts and candy.

The problem with added sugars is that the added calories they provide might tip you over your daily calorie (energy) requirement. For example, one 12-ounce can of non-diet soda contains 8 teaspoons of sugar, or 130 calories. These are often called empty calories because they provide energy but no other nutrients of any note. Extra calories contribute to the extra pounds that can eventually lead to health problems such as diabetes and obesity. Limiting foods and drinks with added sugars is an easy way to cut calories, thus leaving plenty of room in your calorie budget to enjoy more deliciously nutrient-dense foods—"the foods that love you back," as Dr. David Katz calls them.

What about fruit juice? That's natural.

The problem with fruit juice is that it's all too easy to overdo it on calories because it is rich in natural sugars but, unlike whole fruit, does not contain ▶**fiber** to help fill you up. If you down a large (22 oz/650 ml) orange juice after an intense workout, you will have downed around 240 calories, (1,000 kilojoules)—that's equal to nearly four large oranges. While we would not go as far as to say the natural sugars in juice are "added sugars," we do suggest you keep your intake moderate—one serving (½ cup/120 milliliters) a day when it comes to juice. The same goes for trendy drinks such as coconut water.

WHAT DO DIETARY GUIDELINES SAY ABOUT ADDED SUGARS?

Most countries, including the United States, the United Kingdom, Australia, and New Zealand, have official dietary guidelines that are updated every few years. These guidelines recognize that poor diet choices with extra calories are contributing to obesity and chronic disease. For example, the USDA Dietary Guidelines state: "Americans are experiencing an epidemic of overweight and obesity. Poor diet and physical inactivity also are linked to major causes of illness and death. To correct these problems, many Americans must make significant changes in their eating habits and lifestyles."[50]

To help people make appropriate changes to their diet, the guidelines provide recommendations for healthy eating based on the best available scientific evidence at the time of publication. Although there are differences from one country to another, they typically encourage us to eat plenty of vegetables, legumes, fruits, and grains (including breads, rice, pasta, and noodles, preferably whole-grain); and to include lean meat, fish, poultry, eggs, legumes, nuts, milk, yogurts, cheeses, and/or alternatives (low-fat where possible) in our diets. And they recommend that we limit added sugar, along with salt, saturated fats, and alcohol; that we drink plenty of water; and that we be physically active.

United States
The 2010 *Dietary Guidelines for Americans* advise people to "limit the consumption of foods that contain refined grains, especially refined grain foods that contain solid fats, added sugars, and sodium." They go on to make the point that "foods containing solid fats and added sugars are no more likely to contribute to weight gain than any other source of calories in an eating pattern that is within calorie limits." That's the key: "within calorie limits."

Australia
Australia's dietary guidelines published in 2013 advise Australians to "limit intake of foods and drinks containing added sugars such as confectionery, sugar-sweetened soft drinks and cordials, fruit drinks, vitamin waters, energy and sports drinks."

New Zealand
New Zealand's Ministry of Health recommends that people "prepare foods or choose pre-prepared foods, drinks, and snacks . . . with little added sugar; limit your intake of high-sugar foods."

United Kingdom
The United Kingdom's Food Standards Agency states that "the Government recommends that all healthy individuals should consume a diet that contains . . . less saturated fat, salt, and sugar." The agency recommends that no more than 11 percent of calories come from added sugars.

PUTTING A NUMBER ON "LIMITING"
Dietary guidelines generally don't define exactly what they mean by "limiting added sugars" (the UK is an exception to this rule). For that, you can turn to other health organizations.

Currently, the World Health Organization (WHO) recommends that people not eat more than 10 percent of their total energy from added sugars. (For a typical American adult male consuming 2,000 calories a day, for example, this is equal to around 12 teaspoons—200 calories.) This is based on the observation in epidemiological studies that a population has an increased risk of developing tooth decay when its average added-sugar consumption goes above 10 percent of calories. Bacteria in the mouth contribute to tooth decay, and their preferred fuel is sugars, oligosaccharides, and starches.

The American Heart Association recommends a lower threshold: "On the basis of the 2005 U.S. Dietary Guidelines, intake of added sugars greatly exceeds discretionary calorie allowances [your treat foods], regardless of energy needs. In view of these considerations, the American Heart Association recommends reductions in the intake of added sugars. A prudent upper limit of intake is half of the discretionary calorie allowance, which for most American women is no more than 100 calories (6 teaspoons) per day and for most American men is no more than 150 calories (9 teaspoons) per day from added sugars."[51]

As of March 2014, the WHO's new draft guidelines suggest further reductions, recommending that consuming less than 5 percent of total calories from added sugars may provide additional health benefits.

On February 28, 2014, Michelle Obama formally announced the proposed food label changes that are central to her signature Let's Move campaign. The proposed changes include listing not only the amount of total sugar, but also how much *added* sugar is in a serving. This will certainly be helpful for consumers wanting to keep their added-sugar intake within the recommended guidelines.

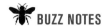 **BUZZ NOTES**

What do 5 percent and 10 percent added sugars look like in an overall healthy 2,000-calorie (8,000-kilojoule) diet?

5 percent added sugars looks like this (sources of sugar appear in red):

BREAKFAST	LUNCH	DINNER
⅔ cup rolled oats	2 slices of hearty whole-grain bread	2 ounces (60 g) beef strips
1 cup reduced-fat (1–2%) milk	2 teaspoons olive oil margarine	1½ cups Asian-style stir-fry noodles
2 teaspoons wildflower honey	3½ ounces (100 g) canned red salmon	2 cups Asian-style stir-fry vegetables
½ grapefruit	½ cup mixed salad (lettuce, cucumber, and tomato)	1 tablespoon sesame oil
	One 7-ounce (200 g) container plain yogurt	¼ cup Asian stir-fry sauce
	½ banana	Small glass (100 ml) white wine
		½ cup reduced-fat vanilla ice cream
		½ cup strawberries

2,000 calories; 106 g protein; 60 g fat; 15 g saturated fat; 160 mg cholesterol; 228 g total carbohydrate; 82 g total sugars; 25 g added sugars; 25 g fiber; 1,765 mg sodium

10 percent added sugars looks like this:

BREAKFAST	LUNCH	DINNER
⅔ cup rolled oats	2 slices of hearty whole-grain bread	2 ounces (60 g) beef strips
1 cup reduced-fat (1–2%) milk	2 teaspoons olive oil margarine	1½ cups Asian-style stir-fry noodles
1 tablespoon (3 teaspoons) wildflower honey	3½ ounces (100 g) canned red salmon	2 cups Asian-style stir-fry vegetables
½ grapefruit	½ cup mixed salad (lettuce, cucumber, and tomato)	1 tablespoon sesame oil
	One 7-ounce (200 g) container low-fat vanilla yogurt	¼ cup Asian stir-fry sauce
	½ banana	½ cup reduced-fat vanilla ice cream
		½ cup strawberries
		1 piece (8 g) milk chocolate

2,040 calories; 105 g protein; 62 g fat; 16 g saturated fat; 162 mg cholesterol; 250 g total carbohydrate; 104 g total sugars; 50 g added sugars; 25 g fiber; 1,742 mg sodium

WHAT DOES THE US ACADEMY OF NUTRITION AND DIETETICS SAY ABOUT SUGARS AND SWEETENERS?

In 2012, the Academy of Nutrition and Dietetics published a comprehensive, research-based position statement on sugars and sweeteners. It says: "Consumers can safely enjoy a range of nutritive sweeteners and nonnutritive sweeteners (NNS) when consumed within an eating plan that is guided by current federal nutrition recommendations, such as the Dietary Guidelines for Americans and the Dietary Reference Intakes, as well as individual health goals and personal preference."

The statement makes a point of noting that "a preference for sweet taste is innate, and sweeteners can increase the pleasure of eating." With respect to specific kinds of sweeteners, it states:

Nutritive sweeteners contain carbohydrate and provide energy. They occur naturally in foods or may be added in food processing or by consumers before consumption. Higher intake of added sugars is associated with higher energy intake and lower diet quality, which can increase the risk for obesity, prediabetes, type 2 diabetes, and cardiovascular disease. Polyols (also referred to as sugar alcohols) add sweetness with less energy and may reduce risk for dental caries. Foods containing polyols and/or no added sugars can, within food labeling guidelines, be labeled as sugar-free. NNS are those that sweeten with minimal or no carbohydrate or energy. They are regulated by the Food and Drug Administration as food additives or generally recognized as safe. The Food and Drug Administration approval process includes determination of probable intake, cumulative effect from all uses, and toxicology studies in animals. Seven NNS are approved for use in the United States: acesulfame K, aspartame, luo han guo fruit extract, neotame, saccharin, stevia, and sucralose. They have different functional properties that may affect perceived taste or use in different food applications. All NNS approved for use in the United States are determined to be safe. [Since this statement was published, an eighth NNS has been approved by the FDA in May 2014: advantame.]

THE ULTIMATE GUIDE TO SUGARS & SWEETENERS

They also offer practical suggestions for healthfully consuming ▶**nutritive** and ▶**nonnutritive sweeteners**:

- Cut back on calorie-containing sweeteners by drinking fewer sugar-sweetened beverages, sports or fruit drinks.
- Decrease consumption of foods that are high in added sugars, such as sugar-sweetened beverages or grain-based desserts, including cakes, cookies, and pastries.
- Enjoy the sweet taste of foods and beverages, but keep your calorie count lower by choosing from the variety of no-calorie sweeteners approved for use by the Food and Drug Administration.
- As part of a healthful eating plan as outlined in the 2010 Dietary Guidelines for Americans, safely enjoy the range of calorie-containing and no-calorie sweeteners in foods and beverages.[52]

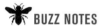 **BUZZ NOTES**

The Food Culprit Problem

In a thoughtful piece in *The New York Times*, "Unhappy Meals," Michael Pollan documents the "shift from eating food to eating nutrients" and argues that relying solely on information regarding individual nutrients has led people and policy makers to make poor decisions about food and nutrition over the last forty years.[53]

The low-fat story is a good example of this type of "nutritionism" at work. Research from the 1960s and 1970s linking high-fat diets (especially saturated fat) with cardiovascular disease led to widespread government health recommendations to cut back on fat intake—a mantra quickly enshrined in dietary guidelines the world over to beat heart disease and the "battle of the bulge." The food industry responded by developing a vast array of reduced- and low-fat alternatives (often substituting refined ▶**carbohydrates** for the fat). People responded, too, cutting back on full-fat products and chowing down on the "diet" and "lite" alternatives with gusto. And although heart-health statistics improved, the scales told a different story. People just kept on getting fatter. Why? Well, what you replace fat with really does matter.

The huge success of Dr. Atkins's *New Diet Revolution*, with his message that excessive *carbohydrate* consumption (not fat, saturated or otherwise) was the bad guy behind the US obesity epidemic, shined the spotlight back onto carbohydrates in general. Since the Atkins Revolution, one carbohydrate in particular—▶**fructose**—has been singled out as the cause of the US obesity epidemic, especially in the form of ▶**high fructose corn syrups (HFCS)** used in increasing amounts by the US food industry from the late 1970s. The parallel increase in rates of overweight and obesity with the increasing use of HFCS has led some researchers to believe that fructose is, in fact, a major cause of the obesity epidemic. Yet rates of overweight and obesity have increased around the globe, even in countries such as Australia, where HFCS is not used in food and beverage production.

In Australia, the United Kingdom, and the United States, per capita consumption of refined ▶**granulated sugar** (▶sucrose) decreased by 23 percent, 10 percent, and 20 percent respectively from 1980 to 2003. However, when all sources of ▶**nutritive sweeteners**, including HFCS, were considered, per capita consumption decreased in Australia (16 percent) and the United Kingdom (5 percent) but increased in the United States (23 percent). During this period, the prevalence of obesity increased threefold in Australia and at least doubled in the United Kingdom. So, while excessive consumption of fructose in the form of HFCS may be a contributing factor to the US obesity epidemic, it seems unlikely that it is a major cause elsewhere.

It appears that, in Australia, at least, people took the message to eat less sugar very seriously. (Australians are very good at adopting public health messages: Australia has one of the lowest rates of cigarette smoking in the world due to decades of the Quit campaign, and the Slip, Slop, Slap campaign to reduce sun exposure has been so successful that rates of vitamin D deficiency are skyrocketing.)

Maybe the real problem is that, while we focus on finding a key culprit to blame for the obesity epidemic and obsessively counting the grams of fat or sugar we consume, we inadvertently consume more food and drink overall. Also, we often overlook the fact that most of us are much less physically active than people were a few decades ago.

Foods and traditional ways of eating it involve far more than nutrients. Food is one of life's great pleasures to be enjoyed with family and friends. It is part of our cultural heritage and, for many people, integral to religious beliefs. If we want to deal with the current obesity epidemic without totally destroying our enjoyment of food and life, we must learn to enjoy mealtimes and meals built around whole foods.

BRAZIL'S NEW DIETARY GUIDELINES FOCUS ON FOOD AND THE ENJOYMENT OF MEALS

Early in 2014, the federal Ministry of Health of Brazil issued the final draft of a new guide to food, nutrition, and the enjoyment of healthy meals. It takes a broad and comprehensive view of health, including the social, cultural, economic, and environmental dimensions of food systems and supplies and dietary patterns. In particular it examines the central role of different types of processing on food quality. The review process may change the final guidelines, but we found these draft guidelines inspiring, with their big-picture approach and their focus on enjoying good food and meals rather than checking off a nutrient to-do list. The ten main recommendations are:

1. Prepare meals from staple and fresh foods.
2. Use oils, fats, sugar, and salt in moderation.
3. Limit consumption of ready-to-consume food and drink products.
4. Eat regular meals, paying attention, and in appropriate environments.
5. Eat in company whenever possible.
6. Buy food at places that offer varieties of fresh foods. Avoid those that mainly sell products ready for consumption.
7. Develop, practice, share, and enjoy your skills in food preparation and cooking.
8. Plan your time to give meals and eating proper time and space.
9. When you eat out, choose restaurants that serve freshly made dishes and meals. Avoid fast food chains.
10. Be critical of the commercial advertisement of food products.[54]

ADDING REFINED STARCH AND MALTODEXTRINS ADDS CALORIES, TOO

In their rush to condemn added sugar, everyone seems to have forgotten about the other forms of ▶carbohydrates that we eat: ▶starches and ▶maltodextrins. Here we are talking about refined starches such as cornstarch, not starch as it is found in traditional, nutrient-rich foods such as root vegetables, legumes, wheat, brown rice, pearl barley, quinoa, and rolled oats.

It's easy to understand why refined starches and maltodextrins are invisible:

- They are not listed in the Nutrition Information/Nutrition Facts panel on foods.
- The names for added refined starches and maltodextrins are often unpronounceable, such as acetylated distarch phosphate (or food additive code number 1414, if you prefer).

Why does it matter? Refined starches and maltodextrins contain essentially the same amount of calories (kilojoules), total carbohydrates, and fiber as do refined sugars and, without fortification, are just as devoid of vitamins and minerals. They also have a high glycemic index. In a nutshell, refined starches and maltodextrins can be as detrimental to our health as added refined sugar.

SUGARS, SWEETENERS, AND DIGESTION

WHAT HAPPENS WHEN WE EAT FOODS CONTAINING CALORIC SUGARS AND SWEETENERS?

Regardless of their source, most of the ▶**carbohydrates** in foods that we eat are digested in the stomach and small intestine, absorbed into the bloodstream, and, one way or another, converted to the sugar ▶**glucose**. This includes all ▶**starches**, ▶**maltodextrins**, and most sugars. Here's how your body does this:

For most carbohydrates the process is relatively simple. Starches and ▶**oligosaccharides** are simply chains of glucose. Small proteins (known as enzymes) called amylases found in saliva and intestinal digestive juices (secreted from the pancreas) snip each bond between the glucose molecules, so that by the end of the digestive process you wind up with pure glucose in the small intestine, which is then actively transported through the intestinal wall into the bloodstream.

Sugars are a little more complicated. In order to be absorbed into the bloodstream, the common ▶**disaccharides** ▶**maltose**, ▶**lactose**, and ▶**sucrose** need to be broken down into their constituent ▶**monosaccharides** (single sugars). Like starches and maltodextrins, this is done by specific enzymes in our small intestine:

- Maltose is very quickly broken down by the enzyme maltase into two glucose molecules (single units of glucose), which are transported straight into the bloodstream.
- Sucrose is broken down into its constituent glucose and ▶**fructose** molecules (single units of fructose) by the enzyme sucrase.
- Lactose is broken down to glucose and ▶**galactose** molecules (single units of galactose) by the enzyme lactase (except in those who are lactose intolerant).

The glucose, fructose, and galactose molecules are then absorbed into the bloodstream.

The glucose molecules (we will shorten this to "glucose" from here on) circulate throughout the body and can be absorbed directly into the cells of most of the body's tissues and organs, where it usually ends up as pyruvate and adenosine triphosphate (ATP), which is our body's main energy currency. Normally, pyruvate is also converted to ATP, thus producing more energy.

Galactose and fructose molecules, however, go to the liver for further processing. Here it gets rather technical, but we have simplified as much as we can. In the liver, fructose is rapidly removed from the bloodstream, phosphor is added to the fructose, and the resulting phosphorylated fructose enters what is known scientifically as the glycolytic pathway, where, through a series of chemical reactions, it usually ends up as pyruvate and ATP. Similarly, galactose is extracted from the blood and converted to glucose in the liver, and again converted to pyruvate and ATP, just like glucose.

The release of these alternate fuels (e.g., glucose, pyruvate) into the bloodstream depends on your energy balance. For example, if your body's energy stores are low after an overnight fast (which typically occurs when we are sleeping!), the liver will release glucose from its glycogen (see page 77) stores to keep the brain, nervous system, and other vital organs functioning. However, just after a meal, the liver will store these fuels (typically as glycogen) for use later. Also, all single sugars (monosaccharides) can be converted to fat (triglycerides) in the liver through a series of complex chemical reactions. The fat can either be stored for later use or released into the bloodstream, depending on the body's requirements. Fructose is converted more readily than the other monosaccharides, and when consumed in large amounts (more than 50 grams of pure fructose in one "dose"), it will raise blood triglyceride levels. However, most people do not eat large amounts of pure fructose in one sitting!

When glucose enters the bloodstream, the pancreas releases the hormone insulin, which signals most of the body's organs and tissues to absorb the glucose from the blood. People with diabetes produce either no insulin (type 1) or not enough insulin (type 2), and this is why their ▶**blood glucose** levels rise too high after consuming a high-carbohydrate meal or drink.

What happens to the fructose? It depends. We use most of it for energy, and under normal circumstances, very little is stored as fat. A recent review of the scientific evidence found that our bodies:

- Use up 45 percent of pure fructose (that's fructose consumed on its own, such as Fruisana—pure crystalline fructose) within 3 to 6 hours for energy
- Use up 66 percent of fructose consumed with glucose (as it typically is in nature, such as sucrose, or table sugar) within 3 to 6 hours for energy
- Convert roughly a third (29 percent) to a half (54 percent) of all fructose we consume to glucose
- Seem to convert less than 1 percent of fructose directly to blood fat (triglycerides).[55]

WHAT HAPPENS WHEN WE EAT FOODS CONTAINING POLYOLS (SUGAR ALCOHOLS)?

Most ▶**polyols**, such as ▶**sorbitol**, ▶**erythritol**, and ▶**xylitol**, are poorly absorbed in our intestines. That's why they provide fewer calories than sugars and other sweeteners and have little effect on ▶**blood glucose** levels. For example, ▶**lactitol** is very poorly absorbed by the body in the small intestine, while most (up to 90 percent) of erythritol is rapidly absorbed and excreted in urine. Most of the others travel in the bloodstream to the liver, where they are eventually converted to ▶**glucose**, pyruvate, and ATP, just like regular sugars.

As polyols pass through the digestive tract, they bind water along the way. Bacteria in the large intestine can use polyols for fuel. Breakdown products when the bacteria metabolize polyols include gas and short-chain fatty acids, which also attract water. Depending on the type of ▶**sugar alcohol**, how much you consume, and the bacteria in your large intestine (we are all different), you may experience some degree of gas, bloating, and possibly even diarrhea. This is why foods that contain a certain amount of polyols (10 to 25 grams of polyol per 100 grams of the food) are required to provide a warning statement that they "may have a laxative effect."

WHERE DO THE GLYCEMIC INDEX (GI) AND GLYCEMIC LOAD (GL) FIT INTO THE DIGESTIVE PICTURE?

The glycemic index, or GI, is simply a relative ranking that gives us an indication of how fast our body is going to digest, absorb, and metabolize ▶**carbohydrate** foods and convert them to ▶**glucose**. The ranking is based on testing each food in healthy people, not in test tubes (see below). Pure glucose, which is digested and absorbed in a flash, is given a value of 100, and all other carbohydrates are ranked against this. Some foods break down quickly during digestion ("gushers," with a glycemic index of 70 or above), and the glucose in our blood increases rapidly; others break down slowly during digestion, and the glucose is released gradually into the blood ("tricklers," with a glycemic index of 55 or below). And, of course, there are the moderates in between. The glycemic index is simply the measure that tells us which food will do what.

HOW THE GI IS MEASURED

The glycemic index of specific foods is measured in a small group of healthy adults (typically ten or more people) following an internationally standardized procedure. Each volunteer is given a 50-gram (usually) portion of available carbohydrate ("available" basically means it doesn't include dietary ▶**fiber**); then their ▶**blood glucose** levels are measured and plotted every thirty minutes for the following two hours. This process is followed for both the standard food (usually glucose) and the test food, so there are two separate test stages.

STEP 1: On the first day, the volunteers are given a 50-gram portion of glucose, and their blood glucose levels are measured every 30 minutes for 2 hours.

STEP 2: On the second day (usually a couple of days later), they are given a serving of a test food that contains 50 grams of available carbohydrate, and again their blood glucose levels are measured every 30 minutes for 2 hours.

STEP 3: The blood glucose levels from both days are then plotted on a graph, the dots are joined to create a blood glucose curve, and the area below the blood glucose curve is calculated using computer software. The area below the curve for the test food is divided by the area below the curve for pure glucose to derive the glycemic index, which is simply a percentage.

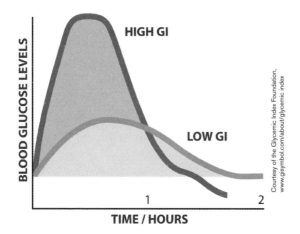

Courtesy of the Glycemic Index Foundation, www.gisymbol.com/about/glycemic index

The glycemic index is such an important part of understanding sugars and sweeteners that we've put a good deal of information on it right at the start of the book. See page 12 or the University of Sydney's glycemic index website (glycemicindex.com) for more information.

ADDITIONAL HEALTH ISSUES

TOOTH DECAY

Highly fermentable ▶**carbohydrates** in the form of sugars, ▶**oligosaccharides** (chains of three to ten sugars), and ▶**starches** can all contribute to tooth decay (cavities/dental caries). Overall, sugars appear to be more cariogenic (that means "likely to promote tooth decay") than oligosaccharides and starches, with the exception of ▶**lactose**.

Whether or not a sugary food or drink will cause tooth decay depends on a wide range of factors including:

- How much and how often you consume the food or drink
- The food's acidity and its buffering power (that's the food's ability to minimize the overall acidity)
- The food's consistency (texture) and its retention in your mouth
- Your overall eating and drinking pattern (i.e., how much and how often you eat and drink).

In addition, your susceptibility to developing tooth decay depends on your oral microflora (mouth bacteria), the flow rate and composition of your saliva, and whether or not you live in an area that has a fluoridated water supply and/or use a fluoride toothpaste.

Consuming added sugars and foods high in added sugars frequently is clearly associated with an increased risk of developing dental caries, independent of the actual amount you eat or drink. So rather than nibble or sip on them throughout the day, you are probably better off downing them in a single sitting and then brushing your teeth with a fluoride toothpaste.

▶**Polyols** (▶**sugar alcohols**) are not well fermented by oral bacteria, nor do they have the acidifying impact on plaque that most sugars do. Thus, unlike other ▶**nutritive sweeteners**, they generally do not promote tooth decay.

Some studies have even suggested that ▶**xylitol** may be anti-cariogenic (helps prevent tooth decay), as it has antibacterial properties that act on some of the fermenting bacteria found in plaque. There is evidence suggesting that between 2.9 and 10.7 grams of xylitol per day will significantly decrease tooth decay.[56] It is, however, important to note that the majority of research into the anticariogenic properties of polyols has been conducted either in test tubes or with chewing gums, lozenges/tablets, and mouthwash. It is therefore difficult to say whether they work the same way when added to other foods.

▶**Nonnutritive sweeteners (NNS)** such as ▶**sucralose** are also not well fermented by oral bacteria, nor do they have the acidifying impact on plaque that most sugars do. So, generally they do not promote tooth decay. However, it comes down to how they are used. For example, "diet" soft drinks that contain NNS are acidic, which means they can still, in theory, contribute to dental erosion. In addition, because they are usually so sweet, most NNS are diluted and bulked up for tabletop use. The bulking agent is frequently ▶**maltodextrins**, which can be used as a fuel by oral bacteria. So, in theory, some non-nutritive tabletop sweeteners may contribute to tooth decay.

DIABETES AND SUGAR

There are two types of diabetes: Type 1 diabetes is an autoimmune condition triggered by unknown environmental factors. Type 2 diabetes is largely inherited, but lifestyle factors such as a lack of exercise or being overweight or obese increase the risk of developing it.

While diabetes is by definition a condition characterized by too much sugar in the blood, that sugar is ▶**glucose**, which comes from the sugars, ▶**oligosaccharides**, and ▶**starches** found in a broad range of ▶**carbohydrate**-containing foods and drinks.

Foods that produce high ▶**blood glucose** levels (BGLs) are associated with an increased risk of type 2 diabetes, but on average sugars have a more moderate effect on BGLs than starches. The total amount of carbohydrate that you consume, and the speed of its digestion as described by its glycemic index, are the strongest predictors of the effect of any given food or drink on your blood glucose levels.

People with diabetes don't simply need to restrict or avoid sugars to manage their blood glucose levels. They need to consider all the available carbohydrates in food: the sugars, ▶**maltodextrins**, and starches. It's the total carbohydrate that matters, not the sugars alone. Based on this, the world's leading diabetes associations, including the American Diabetes Association, the Canadian Diabetes Association, and Diabetes UK agree that:

- Sugar does not cause diabetes.
- Sugar-free diets are not recommended to people living with diabetes.

How we know that eating too much sugar does not cause diabetes

We know from the findings of observational studies from around the world in which large groups of people have a medical checkup, their dietary patterns are measured, and they are followed up with regularly for long periods of time (e.g., five to twenty years) that there is either no association or a negative association between total sugar intake, the commonly consumed ▶**monosaccharides** and ▶**disaccharides**, and risk of developing type 2 diabetes. The only exception is ▶**fructose**, for which two studies show no association and two show a positive association.[57]

On the other hand, the findings from observational studies do suggest that excessive consumption of sugar-sweetened beverages (more than one or two 12-ounce/360-ml drinks a day) is associated with an increased risk of developing type 2 diabetes.[58] Surprisingly, there is also evidence linking "diet" soft drinks with the development of type 2 diabetes.

Unlike randomized controlled trials, observational studies do not prove cause and effect (causality); consequently, more research is needed to determine if these associations are real. It could be that people usually drink regular or diet soft drinks with other highly processed foods (chips, French fries, savory snacks, pastries, etc.) or alcohol, and that it's the overall dietary pattern of highly refined carbohydrates along with a poor diet in general that's really to blame. There is also the matter of thirst. One of the classic signs of diabetes is incredible thirst. Cold beverages quench thirst better than hot beverages, such as tea and coffee. So it may be what we call reverse causality—people are drinking more cold beverages (water, diet, and regular soft drinks) because they have higher than normal blood glucose levels.

Fortunately, there have, in fact, been a number of randomized controlled trials that involved consumption of a healthy diet and regular physical activity by large groups of people for long periods of time that have proven that you can prevent, or at the very least delay the onset of, type 2 diabetes. Therefore, these studies also prove the reverse: that poor diet and physical inactivity can contribute to the risk of developing type 2 diabetes, or increase your chances of developing it earlier if you are genetically predisposed to the condition. Systematic reviews of these randomized controlled trials suggest that the best way to reduce the risk of developing type 2 diabetes is to consume 500 to 600 fewer calories (2,000 to 2,500 fewer kilojoules) each day by eating less fat, and in particular to reduce intake of saturated fat and increase intake of dietary ▶**fiber**.

Of course, some people may also reduce their caloric intake by reducing the amount of added sugars they consume, although this was not a specific goal of these particular studies.[59]

"Diabetic-friendly" foods

The food industry sometimes identifies foods as "diabetic" or "diabetic-friendly" as part of their marketing strategy. So-called "diabetic" or "diabetic-friendly" foods are typically processed food products sweetened with a range of sugar substitutes—▶**nutritive sweeteners** such as ▶**maltitol**, ▶**mannitol**, ▶**xylitol**, and **nonnutritive sweeteners** such as ▶**aspartame**, ▶**sucralose**, and ▶**stevia** or with blends of these. With careful formulation the manufacturers can make these products taste much the same as the regular sugar-sweetened alternatives. Some of these foods and beverages do contain fewer calories and/or carbohydrates than their counterparts, but most of the time they are very similar in total grams of carbohydrate and lower only in sugar (▶**sucrose**). They usually cost more and may include additives, such as ▶**polyols**, that can cause side effects of gas, bloating, and diarrhea if consumed in excess. People with diabetes eat the same foods as people without diabetes. A "real" diabetic-friendly food is a naturally healthy whole food, high in ▶**fiber**, slow to digest, allowing a slower insulin response. Examples of healthy foods include fresh fruits, vegetables, whole grains, legumes (beans), and low-fat dairy products.

Are "diabetic-friendly" foods better for people with diabetes?

Not necessarily. Just because a processed food product is low in sugar or contains no added sugar does not automatically make it a healthy choice. Sugar-free or reduced-sugar cookies, cakes, ice cream, chocolate, and candy should still be saved for special occasions. In fact, some of these foods are still high in calories, saturated fat, and highly refined, high-GI starches, so they will still contribute to weight gain and elevated blood cholesterol and blood glucose levels just as their regular special-occasion counterparts do if eaten too often or in excess.

The 2008 food and nutrition position statement from the American Diabetes Association says that "intake of sucrose and sucrose-containing foods by people with diabetes does not need to be restricted because of concern about aggravating hyperglycemia [high blood glucose]. Sucrose can be substituted for other carbohydrate sources in the meal plan or, if added to the meal plan, adequately covered with insulin or another glucose-lowering medication."[60] We agree. We think it makes much more sense to eat a small amount of traditionally sweetened food on an occasional basis and enjoy its full flavor and texture than to consume poorer-quality substitutes on a regular basis.

We tend to stick with Michael Pollan's key food rules: "Don't eat anything your great-grandmother wouldn't recognize as food. . . . Avoid food products containing ingredients no ordinary human would keep in the pantry. . . . Avoid food products containing ingredients a third-grader cannot pronounce."[61]

Why going on a "sugar-free" diet is not recommended for people living with diabetes

Sugars, oligosaccharides, and starches are digested, absorbed, and metabolized into the sugar glucose, which is, as we have explained, the body's form of energy. Therefore, people with diabetes need to carefully balance the amounts and type of all sugars, oligosaccharides, and starches they eat and drink each day with exercise and diabetes medication (if needed) to ensure their blood glucose levels do not go too high or too low. Simply avoiding sugar does not help people achieve optimal blood glucose levels. Information about the total amount of carbohydrates in a food is available on most food and drink labels.

The International Diabetes Federation recommends that people with diabetes use the glycemic index for assessing the type of carbohydrates they consume. See your registered/accredited dietitian for personalized advice.

 Where can I find GI values?

The best place to check for GI values is the website run by the University of Sydney: glycemicindex.com. In the United States and Australia there are also annual editions of *The Low GI Shopper's Guide to GI Values* available both as print books and e-books, and in Australia the GI value is on the label of some foods. We have also seen apps for GI values, but, sadly, they don't appear to be accurate.

Carbohydrate portions and exchanges explained

Some people with diabetes use the carbohydrate portion or exchange system to help them manage their blood glucose levels. A carbohydrate portion or exchange is an amount of food typically containing 10 or 15 grams of carbohydrates, respectively. The aim of this system is to promote consistency in the amount of carbohydrates eaten from day to day. The emphasis is on carbohydrate quantity. The system assumes that each carbohydrate exchange has the same blood glucose raising effect.

We have put this table together to compare the blood glucose raising effect of 10- and 15-gram carbohydrate portions and exchanges of some typical sugars and sweeteners that have been tested following the international standard method. The GL (glycemic load) columns clearly show that ▶**rice syrup**, a fructose-free sweetener, will have a greater impact on your blood glucose level (BGL) than ▶**regular sugar** or ▶**honey**. We added the energy columns to remind you how quickly calories add up, just a teaspoon at a time.

	GI	GL 2 TEASPOONS (10 GRAMS AVAILABLE CARBOHYDRATES)	CALORIES/KJ 2 TEASPOONS	GL 1 TABLESPOON* (15 GRAMS AVAILABLE CARBOHYDRATES)	CALORIES/KJ 1 TABLESPOON (15 ML, 3 TEASPOONS)
Agave nectar	19–28	2–3	42 calories 176 kJ	3–4	63 calories 264 kJ
Coconut sugar	54	6	32 calories 134 kJ	9	48 calories 202 kJ
Corn syrup	90	9	32 calories 134 kJ	13	48 calories 202 kJ
Fructose	19	?	32 calories 134 kJ	3	48 calories 202 kJ
Glucose	100	10	32 calories 134 kJ	15	48 calories 202 kJ
Golden syrup	63	6	32 calories 134 kJ	9	48 calories 202 kJ
Granulated sugar	65 (avg.)	6	32 calories 134 kJ	9	48 calories 202 kJ
Honey	35–64	4–6	45 calories 190 kJ	6–9	68 calories 280 kJ
Maple syrup	54	6	32 calories 134 kJ	9	48 calories 202 kJ
Molasses (treacle)	68	7	32 calories 134 kJ	10	48 calories 202 kJ
Rice syrup	98	10	32 calories 134 kJ	15	48 calories 202 kJ

*This is the standard 15 ml tablespoon equal to 3 teaspoons.

HYPOGLYCEMIA

Many people who have diabetes and are treating it with medication have firsthand experience of hypoglycemia or low ▶blood glucose (sugar). This is why they carefully monitor their insulin and blood glucose levels to keep things in balance. Blood glucose is considered low when it drops below 70 mg/dL (4 mmol/L). When this happens, people with diabetes need to immediately consume something that provides a readily absorbed form of ▶carbohydrates, such as candy, ▶glucose tablets, soft drinks, or fruit juice/drinks. Kosher Americans use a candy called "Winkies," and others often use jelly beans, Life Savers, Starburst, or Skittles.

Our body needs to maintain a minimum threshold level of glucose in the blood at all times to keep our brain and central nervous system functioning. If for some reason blood glucose levels fall below the threshold and the brain and central nervous system are not getting enough glucose, the result is hypoglycemia, with unpleasant symptoms such as anxiety, trembling, sweating, palpitations, dizziness, and nausea. Poor concentration, drowsiness, and lack of coordination may also be experienced.

If you don't have diabetes but do have vague health problems such as fatigue and depression and think you may have hypoglycemia (or someone tells you that you probably have "low blood sugar"), see your doctor for a proper diagnosis. It is possible you may have reactive, or rebound, hypoglycemia. This occurs after eating and is the most common form of hypoglycemia. When blood glucose levels rise too quickly after eating, they cause an excessive amount of insulin to be released. This draws too much glucose out of the blood and causes blood glucose levels to fall quickly, often to below normal. The result is what is called reactive hypoglycemia. (See Buzz Notes, below).

As having an irregular eating pattern is the most common dietary habit seen in people who have reactive hypoglycemia, it is important to consult a dietitian and put together an appropriate eating plan. If your blood glucose level can be prevented from rising too quickly, then your pancreas will not produce excessive, unnecessary amounts of insulin, which will cause your blood glucose levels to plunge to abnormally low levels. Many people achieve smooth, steady blood glucose levels by switching from high-GI foods to low-GI foods. To help prevent reactive hypoglycemia it is important to:

- Eat regular meals (and snacks, as well, if you need them).
- Include low-GI foods in meals and for snacks (e.g., a small container of yogurt or an apple).

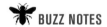 **BUZZ NOTES**
Diagnosing Reactive Hypoglycemia
The diagnosis of reactive hypoglycemia cannot be made simply on the basis of symptoms. Instead, it requires the detection of low ▶**blood glucose** levels when the symptoms are actually being experienced. A blood test is required to do this—a home blood glucose meter is not considered precise enough for the diagnosis of reactive hypoglycemia in people without diabetes.

Because it may be difficult–or almost impossible–for someone to be in the right place at the right time to have a blood sample taken while experiencing the symptoms, a ▶**glucose** tolerance (GTT) test is sometimes used to try to make the diagnosis. This involves drinking pure glucose, which causes the blood glucose levels to rise. If too much insulin is produced in response, a person with reactive hypoglycemia will experience an excessive fall in their blood glucose level. It sounds simple enough, but there are pitfalls. Testing must be done under strictly controlled conditions; low blood glucose is best demonstrated by measuring properly collected blood samples. If your doctor uses an oral glucose tolerance test to diagnose hypoglycemia, you have to continue it for at least three to four hours (the normal time is two hours). Your insulin levels would be measured at the same time.

A few fast facts about hypoglycemia:

■ Hypoglycemia is far less common than once was thought (unless you have diabetes).

■ Hypoglycemia due to a serious medical problem is rare. However, such conditions require in-depth investigation and treatment of the underlying medical problem causing them.

■ Hypoglycemia can often be avoided by eating small amounts of food every 3 to 4 hours instead of going long periods without eating.

HEART DISEASE

People with diabetes have a much higher risk of developing heart disease. The reasons for this are complex and are tied to the typical combination of high blood pressure and abnormal blood fats (cholesterol and triglycerides) that also accompany high ▶**blood glucose** levels. People with pre-diabetes, who have higher than normal blood glucose levels, also have a higher risk of developing heart disease. So it seems logical to conclude that elevated blood glucose levels are a risk factor for heart disease.

Overall, evidence is mounting that the amount and type of ▶**carbohydrates** (sugars and ▶**starches**) that you consume does affect your risk of heart disease. Here is a summary of the key studies that have led to this conclusion:

As of February 2014, three observational studies from the United States suggest that a high consumption of added sugar (15 percent of total calories/kilojoules), typically as sugar-sweetened beverages, can increase the risk of a heart attack.

There is also evidence from a systematic review of randomized controlled trials in people (not animals) that consuming more than 50 grams of crystalline or pure ▶**fructose** a day will raise blood triglycerides—a known heart disease risk factor.

In addition, a systematic review of ten observational studies published in 2012 has found that high-GI diets are associated with heart disease in women.

Similarly, a systematic review of randomized controlled trials in men and women found that a high-GI diet will raise LDL ("bad") cholesterol levels—a more powerful risk factor for heart disease than triglycerides.[62]

So, based on the evidence, if you are at risk of heart disease for whatever reason, it is probably wise to limit your intake of high-glycemic-index carbohydrates in general, including high-glycemic-index sugars, particularly in liquid form such as ▶**corn syrup** (GI 90) and ▶**rice syrup** (GI 98).

OBESITY

Despite catchy phrases such as "sugar is toxic" and "sweet poison," the scientific evidence does not support the belief that sugars per se are uniquely fattening. However, we do recognize that when people strongly *believe* they are, no scientific evidence will change their mind. For those who are interested, here's what the scientific evidence published in leading, peer-reviewed journals shows:

In 2013, *BMJ* published a systematic review and meta-analysis of thirty randomized controlled trials and thirty eight cohort studies investigating the role of sugars and body weight. It concluded: "The data suggest that the change in body fatness that occurs with modifying intake of sugars results from an alteration in energy balance rather than a physiological or metabolic consequence of monosaccharides or disaccharides." It noted that most of the evidence was based on sugar-sweetened-beverage studies.[63]

Indeed, sugar-sweetened beverages (SSBs) have been singled out in recent times as a significant cause of overweight and obesity in many countries. The jury is still out, because recent systematic reviews on the topic have reached different conclusions:

■ Ten reviews proposed that the consumption of SSBs were positively associated with weight gain.

- Seven reviews concluded that there was insufficient evidence, or no association.

Part of the reason for the discrepancy is whether or not observational studies are included. Because they are not on a par with randomized controlled trials, some scientists refuse to include them. Funding source may be another factor, with authors who have no food-industry connections more likely to find a positive association between soft-drink consumption and weight gain.

Whatever the case, SSBs are the major source (just over a third) of added sugars in the United States, where people drink more SSBs than anywhere else in the world (216 liters per person per year in 2002). The take-home from this is that if you are overweight and you drink SSBs, it makes sense to cut way back. However, what you replace them with matters.

It sounds logical that replacing regular sugars with lower-calorie and lower-▶**carbohydrate** alternatives would help people lose weight and reduce their ▶**blood glucose** levels. Somewhat surprisingly, the jury remains out on this, too. In 2012, the American Heart Association and the American Diabetes Association co-published a systematic review of the evidence and concluded that: "At this time, there are insufficient data to determine conclusively whether the use of NNS (nonnutritive sweeteners) to displace caloric sweeteners in beverages and foods reduces added sugars or carbohydrate intakes, or benefits appetite, energy balance, body weight, or cardiometabolic risk factors."

Interpreting the association between consuming SSBs and ▶**nonnutritive**-sweetened beverages (NNSBs) and overall nutrient intake is complex. It's possible that SSB/NNSB intakes could be a general indicator (or marker) for overall poor nutrition, meaning that people who consume more of them generally have poorer quality diets overall.

It's also possible that soft drinks stimulate the appetite for nonnutritious (AKA junk) foods. One study showed that people who downed more soft drinks also chowed down a higher-overall-glycemic-index diet, possibly featuring large quantities of pizza, fries, and burgers, as other studies have suggested.

The bottom line: no single food or nutrient is going to be the sole cause of overweight, obesity, or associated conditions—it's ever so much more complicated than that!

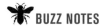

BUZZ NOTES

"The Australian Paradox"

In Australia, rates of overweight and obesity have been rising steadily since the early 1980s, and over the past couple of decades rates of type 2 diabetes have also risen dramatically. This is not surprising, since obesity is a major risk factor for diabetes. In the United States, over a similar time frame, the steadily rising consumption of ▶**high fructose corn syrups** has been linked to increased rates of overweight/obesity and type 2 diabetes.

Given the similarities between the United States and Australia, it's reasonable to assume that similar changes to the food supply may be at the heart of the matter. However, this does not seem to be the case.

Australia is a major producer of ▶**cane sugar** (▶**sucrose**) and not a major producer of corn like the United States. Australians enjoy juicy corn on the cob but consume very little ▶**corn syrup**–high fructose or otherwise–and it is not manufactured domestically. Australians who want to buy corn syrup buy US brands, such as Karo or Aunt Jemima.

Data from the Australian Bureau of Statistics on "apparent consumption" (how much of a particular food or ingredient is available for consumption for a particular population) of sugar shows that the amount of sugar available for human consumption in Australia peaked just after World War II and has been declining slowly ever since, with a few peaks and valleys along the way.

The evidence for a direct role of sugar-sweetened beverages (SSBs) in the development of obesity is very plausible and is growing. There's no arguing with that. But sales of SSBs decreased in Australia between 1997 and 2011, and at the same time the amount of sugar in these beverages was also dropping. The average Australian consumed 9.2 kg of sugar from beverages in 1997 but 7.6 kg in 2011–that's nearly 20 percent less over a fifteen-year period.

Finally, results from Australia's National Nutrition Surveys in 1995 and 2011–2012 show that the amount of total sugars consumed has decreased by about 10 percent, from 112 grams per day to 101 grams per day. (About half of the total sugar consumed by Australians is added sugar.)

The reason sugar consumption is decreasing in Australia is reasonably straightforward. Sweetener surveys conducted by Food Standards Australia and New Zealand in 1994 and 2003 indicate that the use of alternative sweeteners has increased from 51 percent to 66 percent. For people who see themselves as very independent, Australians are unbelievably obedient when it comes to health messages. In droves, they are quitting smoking, covering themselves in sunscreen, and taking vitamin D. They have also cut back on added sugar and sugary foods and switched to alternative sweeteners. Therefore, the body of evidence suggests that in Australia, increased rates of overweight, obesity, and type 2 diabetes are not positively related to reduced consumption of sugars overall. This is what has been termed the Australian Paradox.

What is "apparent consumption" again?

It is a way of working out how much of a particular food or ingredient is available for consumption for a particular population. It is not the same as food or nutrient intake, as a significant proportion of food that is produced or purchased is wasted—up to a third in developed nations, according to some recent estimates. It does provide useful information about long-term trends in a population's consumption of particular foods and ingredients, however.

SPECIAL DIETS

FRUCTOSE MALABSORPTION

Unlike ▶**glucose**, ▶**fructose** is not actively transported into the intestinal wall. Despite this, it is absorbed at a faster rate than would be expected if it was just passively absorbed. While the complete mechanism of fructose absorption in the human intestine is not understood, it is known that it is taken up by glucose transporter 5 (GLUT5).

Lots of people (40 to 80 percent) have fructose malabsorption when they consume fructose on its own in solution (water). Some people can absorb less than 15 grams of fructose, whereas others have trouble completely absorbing 30 to 40 grams. Most of us will suffer from flatulence and diarrhea if we consume 50 grams or more of pure fructose.

It's a completely different story if we consume fructose with glucose or ▶**starch**. Most of us absorb it completely, even people who couldn't absorb it on its own. For example, research shows that when we consume equal amounts of glucose and fructose together (i.e., 50 percent fructose/50 percent glucose, as in ▶**sucrose**), there is no evidence of malabsorption in most adults. There is also little evidence that slightly higher fructose concentrations, such as those commonly found in ▶**high fructose corn syrups** (55 percent fructose/45 percent glucose) cause any appreciable symptoms of malabsorption, either.

Since fructose rarely occurs naturally in the diet in the absence of other carbohydrates, some scientists have suggested that, for most of us, fructose malabsorption is really only a problem in academic studies that provide large amounts of pure fructose by mouth.

FODMAPS

The acronym ▶**FODMAPs** stands for Fermentable Oligosaccharides, Disaccharides, Monosaccharides and Polyols. Recent research has found that avoiding FODMAPs may improve symptoms of irritable bowel syndrome (IBS) in many people.

IBS is a very common gastrointestinal disorder. It is characterized by chronic and relapsing symptoms: lower abdominal pain and discomfort, bloating, gas, distention, and altered bowel habits (ranging from diarrhea to constipation) but with no abnormal pathology in the gut. It's important to note that IBS should only be diagnosed by a medical practitioner and that other illnesses, including inflammatory bowel disease (IBD), celiac disease, and colorectal cancers, be ruled out.

A brief discussion of the acronym will help you to understand what a low-FODMAP diet requires:

- *Fermentable* refers to the process through which bacteria in our large intestine break down undigested ▸**carbohydrate** to produce gases (hydrogen, methane, and carbon dioxide).
- The ▸**oligosaccharides** are classified as dietary ▸**fibers** in most countries and include ▸**fructooligosaccharides** (FOS) found in wheat, rye, onions, and garlic, and galactooligosaccharides (GOS) found in legumes/pulses (dried beans, chickpeas, and lentils), but *not* the more common oligosaccharide, ▸**maltodextrin**.
- The particular ▸**disaccharide** focused on is ▸**lactose**, found in milk, soft cheese, and yogurts, but not the other common disaccharides ▸**sucrose** and ▸**maltose**.
- The ▸**monosaccharide** focused on is ▸**fructose** (in excess of ▸**glucose**, as discussed above).
- The ▸**polyols** include most (but not all) ▸**sugar alcohols** (e.g., ▸**sorbitol**, ▸**mannitol**) found naturally in some fruits and vegetables but in increasingly larger quantities as alternative sweeteners.

A low-FODMAP diet can be trialed for six to eight weeks, ideally with the help of a registered (accredited) dietitian, to see if common IBS symptoms decrease or go away completely. If they do, the dietitian can then help with a systematic reintroduction of FODMAP-containing foods to determine which kinds of carbohydrates are actually causing the symptoms and how much can be tolerated before symptoms develop. It's important to note that strict low-FODMAP diets are used for diagnostic purposes and as such are not designed to be consumed for long periods of time. The goal is to diversify the diet as much as possible without gut symptoms.

GLUTEN AND CELIAC DISEASE

Celiac disease is becoming increasingly common, affecting around 1 in 100 people in Australia and the United Kingdom, and 1 in 133 Americans. More people are being diagnosed with celiac disease due to both better diagnosis rates and a true increase in the incidence of celiac disease for as yet unknown reasons.

The immune systems of people with celiac disease react abnormally to the protein gluten, found in wheat, rye, and barley (and a common contaminant in oats), causing damage to their small intestine. The tiny, fingerlike projections known as villi that line the small intestine become inflamed and flattened—a condition known as villous atrophy. As a consequence, the surface area of the intestine available for the absorption of nutrients is reduced, which can lead to various gastrointestinal and malabsorptive symptoms such as diarrhea and/or constipation, large, bulky, foul stools, unwanted weight loss or poor growth in children, flatulence, abdominal bloating, distention or pain, and anemia. The disease can appear without gastrointestinal symptoms; anemia is the most common presentation in adult-onset celiac disease. Long-term complications can be very serious and include infertility, miscarriage, depression, and dental enamel defects. There is also an increased risk of developing certain forms of cancer, such as lymphoma of the small intestine.

If you have a family history of celiac disease and some or all of the above symptoms, it's important that you don't simply self-diagnose celiac disease and commence a gluten-free diet. Blood tests for celiac disease are available, but the diagnosis can only be confirmed by demonstrating the typical villous atrophy of celiac disease in a small intestine biopsy. This involves an endoscopy—a gastroscopy procedure in which several tiny samples of the small bowel are taken and examined under a microscope. Importantly, you must still be eating gluten regularly before the procedure is performed or you may get a false negative result. Genetic tests are also available but can only be used to rule out the possibility of celiac disease, not confirm a diagnosis, as many people have the genes tied to celiac disease but do not have the disease itself.

A gluten-free diet is currently the only known treatment for celiac disease, and it is lifelong, because people with celiac disease remain sensitive to gluten throughout their life—the condition can never be cured. However, by removing the cause of the disease, a gluten-free diet typically allows the lining of the small intestine to heal and symptoms to resolve. As long as the gluten-free diet is adhered to as strictly as possible, problems arising from celiac disease should not return.

Most pure sugars and sweeteners, such as ▸**fructose**, ▸**glucose**, ▸**sucrose**, ▸**lactose**, etc., are gluten-free, as are pure ▸**polyols** and pure ▸**nonnutritive sweeteners**. ▸**Maltose** is an exception, as it can be derived from a wide range of starchy foods, including gluten-containing grains (often barley). Similarly, ▸**confectioners' sugar** is usually made from sucrose with a little bit of ▸**starch**, and the starch may be from corn (gluten-free, and the most common choice in North America) or from a gluten-containing grain (most often wheat).

There's a potential problem with ▸**high-intensity sweeteners**, because they are usually bulked up with ▸**polyols** and ▸**maltodextrins**. The maltodextrins are typically derived from a cheap source of starch, some of which can be from wheat or other gluten-containing grains. However, most common varieties make a gluten-free declaration.

The bottom line: always read the label, and contact the manufacturer if you are unsure.

GLUTEN SENSITIVITY

There is some evidence pointing to the existence of non-celiac gluten sensitivity (sometimes known as "gluten intolerance"). With this condition, small-intestine biopsy results prove that a patient does not have celiac disease, but when he or she avoids gluten, gastrointestinal and other symptoms generally improve. Though many doctors and researchers around the world believe this condition exists, there are no tests for it, and the evidence is uncertain. In addition, a recent Australian study suggests that people with so-called gluten intolerance may not, in fact, be sensitive to gluten as such. Indeed, their gut symptoms may be due to other dietary factors, in particular, fermentable, poorly absorbed short-chain carbohydrates (▸**FODMAPs**) that are found in a wide range of foods. Rather than avoiding gluten, people with these symptoms may instead benefit from a low-FODMAP diet.

PHENYLALANINE AND PHENYLKETONURIA

Phenylketonuria (PKU) is a rare inherited disorder that increases the levels of phenylalanine in the blood. Classical PKU affects 1 in 10,000 to 20,000 newborns, depending on the country of origin. In the United States, for example, it typically occurs in 1 in 10,000 to 15,000 newborns. Managing PKU means sticking to a low-protein diet, with particular emphasis on avoiding foods high in phenylalanine. Some ▶**nonnutritive sweeteners**, such as ▶**aspartame**, contain phenylalanine and are required to state as much on package labels as a warning to those with PKU. Note that most people do not have PKU and therefore are not adversely affected by phenylalanine.

FOR VEGETARIANS AND VEGANS

▶**Granulated sugar** (▶**sucrose**) can be made from ▶**sugar beet** or ▶**sugarcane**. One of the final steps in cane sugar processing is filtration through activated carbon, a form of charcoal that may be of animal, vegetable, or mineral origin. This step is unnecessary for beet sugar. Over half the sugarcane refineries in the United States use charcoal made from animal bones as their activated carbon source. The charcoal used in this filtering process is far removed from its animal source and is deemed kosher. However, some vegetarians and vegans disagree with this perspective. In the United States, "100% organic sugar" or "100% beet sugar" is thought to be bone-char-free.

Some vegans also choose not to eat ▶**honey**, as it is made by bees.

SWEET TALK ON LABELS

THE REGULATIONS

Packaged foods sold in the United States, Canada, the United Kingdom, Australia, New Zealand, and many other parts of the world provide nutrition information on their labels, including fact-based ingredients lists, nutrition facts/information panels, plus content claims such as "no added sugar" and warning statements about phenylalanine content or the potential side effects of large doses of ▶**polyols**. Laws that govern this nutrition information are prepared by government agencies, such as the U.S. Food and Drug Administration (FDA) or Food Standards Australia New Zealand (FSANZ), and are enforceable. So, while the information provided is rarely perfect, you can generally trust it overall, and you certainly can do something about it if you spot a major problem.

INGREDIENTS LISTS

The ingredients list is a really useful tool for supermarket sleuths who want to work out exactly what is in their foods and drinks. Ingredients must be declared in descending order of ingoing weight. So if a sweetener is the first ingredient in the list, you know that the food or drink contains a relatively large quantity of that ingredient, and if it is last on the list, it contains very little. Simple, really.

In Australia and New Zealand, food companies are also required to list the percentage of key characterizing ingredients in the ingredients list. For example, a honey and vanilla yogurt must state in the ingredients list the percent of ▶**honey** actually included. Finally, ingredients must be listed using either:

- The common name of the ingredient, or
- A name that describes the true nature of the ingredient, or, where applicable,

- A generic name such as "sugar" can be used to describe ▶**white sugar**, white refined sugar, ▶**caster sugar**, castor sugar, loaf sugar, or cube sugar, ▶**icing sugar**, coffee sugar, coffee crystals, ▶**raw sugar.**

NAMES AND NUMBERS OF APPROVED ADDITIVES

E numbers are found on food labels on packaged foods sold within the European Union and Switzerland, the Cooperation Council for the Arab States of the Gulf, and Israel. They are occasionally found on packaging in the United States and Canada on imported European products.

Australia and New Zealand's additive code numbering system is the same as Europe's, without the prefix "E."

In North America, the additive will be listed in the ingredients by name. In the United States, additives approved for use by the FDA are classified as GRAS, meaning Generally Recognized As Safe. Health Canada publishes a List of Permitted Sweeteners, which sets out the authorized food additives used to impart a sweet taste to food.

SWEETENER	EUROPE, SWITZERLAND, AND UK– E NUMBER	AUSTRALIA AND NEW ZEALAND– ADDITIVE CODE NUMBER	USA–GRAS STATUS/FDA APPROVED	CANADA– PERMITTED SWEETENERS
Acesulfame K	E950	950	FDA approved	Permitted
Advantame	E969	Approved	FDA approved	
Alitame	E956	956		
Aspartame	E951	951	FDA approved	Permitted
Aspartame + acesulfame salt	E962	962		
Cyclamate	E952	952		
Erythritol	E968	968	GRAS	Permitted
Glycyrrhizin	E958	958	GRAS	
Isomalt	E953	953	GRAS	Permitted
Lactitol	E966	966	GRAS	Permitted
Maltitol	E965	965	GRAS	Permitted

[Table continues]

SWEETENER	EUROPE, SWITZERLAND, AND UK– E NUMBER	AUSTRALIA AND NEW ZEALAND– ADDITIVE CODE NUMBER	USA–GRAS STATUS/FDA APPROVED	CANADA– PERMITTED SWEETENERS
Mannitol	E421	421	GRAS	Permitted
Monk fruit extract	Approved	Approved	GRAS	Permitted
Neotame	E961	961	FDA approved	Permitted
Saccharin	E954	954		
Sorbitol	E420	420	GRAS	Permitted
Steviol glycosides (stevioside, rebaudioside)	E960	960	GRAS	Permitted
Sucralose	E955	955	FDA approved	Permitted
Thaumatin (flavor enhancer)	E957	957	GRAS	Permitted
Xylitol	E967	967	GRAS	Permitted

NUTRITION PANELS

Nearly all packaged foods must provide nutrition information that includes the amount of total ▶**carbohydrates**, total sugars, and, where a claim is made, ▶**sugar alcohols** (▶**polyols**).

In the United States and Canada this information is provided per standard serving of the product. In Australia and New Zealand it is provided per serving ("serve") and per 100 grams, because serving sizes are not standardized. In the United Kingdom it is provided per 100 grams and sometimes per serving (optional).

Because only total sugars are listed in the nutrition facts/information, you might not know how much is naturally occurring (e.g., from fruits, vegetables, milk, etc.) and how much is added. However, you can use the order and number of added sugars in the ingredients list as a rough guide. Here's how: If a 12-ounce (360-ml) can of regular cola contains 39.8 g of sugars and lists sugar as the first ingredient and no other sweeteners, you know that it is all added sugar.

In the United States and Canada, sugar alcohols (polyols) are listed along with sugars under the "carbohydrate" heading and are included in the total. Some manufacturers also label a food with its "net carbs," calculated by subtracting the amount of sugar alcohols and ▶**fiber** from the total carbohydrate count. In Australia and New Zealand, sugar alcohols are usually listed after sodium and are not counted under total carbohydrate. Needless to say, the system in Australia and New Zealand can lead to some confusion.

Finally, ▶**maltodextrins** are not required to be listed in the nutrition facts/information panel. Combined with their often unpronounceable names, these are the truly hidden form of slightly sweet carbohydrates.

SUGAR CONTENT LABEL CLAIMS

A relatively large number of claims about the sugar content of foods are allowed to be made on food labels. They vary from country to country. Below we list some typical ones, along with examples of approved definitions.

Low sugar

United States: "Low sugar" is not strictly defined, but it must be at least 25 percent less sugar than in the reference (similar) food.

Australia/New Zealand: The food or drink must not contain more sugars than (a) 2.5 grams per 100 ml for liquid food; or (b) 5 grams per 100 grams for solid food

X percent sugar-free

United States: "Sugar-free" must be less than 0.5 gram sugar per serving on the label.

Australia/New Zealand: The food or drink is required to meet the conditions for a nutrition content claim about "low sugar," described above (and also, of course, actually be X percent sugar-free)

Reduced sugar, light, or "lite" (also "reduced in sugar," "sugar reduced," "less sugar")

United States: The information is required on how many grams of sugar have been reduced: for example, from 8 to 6 grams per serving. This claim cannot be made on vitamins, minerals, or any supplements.

Australia/New Zealand: To make this claim, the food or drink is required to contain at least 25 percent less sugars than in the same quantity of a reference (similar) food.

No added sugar (also "unsweetened" and "no added sweeteners")

United States: This is a *fact* statement per the FDA, while "reducing dental caries" is an implied *health claim*. It does not include sugar alcohols.

Australia/New Zealand: The food or drink (a) contains no added sugars; or (b) contains no added concentrated fruit juice or deionized fruit juice.

Unsweetened

Australia: The food or drink must (a) meet the conditions for a nutrition content claim about no added sugar; and (b) contain no ▶**high-intensity sweeteners:** ▶**sorbitol,** ▶**mannitol,** ▶**glycerol,** ▶**xylitol,** ▶**isomalt,** ▶**maltitol syrup,** or ▶**lactitol.**

OTHER HEALTH-RELATED LABEL CLAIMS

In the United States and Australia and New Zealand, a health claim is allowed about good oral hygiene (e.g., "tooth-friendly" or "does not promote tooth decay") on certain foods. For example, candy or chewing gum can make the claim if it contains 0.2 percent or less ▶**starch,** dextrins, ▶**mono-,** ▶**di-** and ▶**oligosaccharides,** or other fermentable ▶**carbohydrates** combined; or if it contains more than 0.2 percent fermentable carbohydrates and does not lower plaque pH below 5.7 by bacterial fermentation during thirty minutes after consumption as measured by the indwelling plaque pH test.

LABEL WARNINGS AND ADVISORY STATEMENTS

The addition of ▶**polyols** (▶**sugar alcohols**) to foods and drinks at a level of 10 to 25 grams per 100 grams, depending on the sweetener, triggers the need for an advisory statement on the label regarding the potential for laxative effects.

Labels on foods and drinks that contain ▶**aspartame** must indicate that the food contains phenylalanine, an amino acid that people who have phenylketonuria (PKU) should not consume. See page 243 for more information on PKU.

PART

3

TEST KITCHEN

SUBSTITUTING SUGARS AND SWEETENERS IN TWO CLASSIC RECIPES

When you start reading labels of the various sugars and sweeteners and sugar substitutes, you will discover that many sugar and sweetener products blithely suggest that you can substitute their product for regular ▶**granulated sugar** in your home cooking and baking. Is it that easy? Will it look and taste the same? We asked Chrissy Freer to help us put some of the most popular alternatives to regular sugar through their baking paces to see how they performed.

Chrissy Freer is a food writer, qualified nutritionist, stylist, and editor whose signature style involves creating delicious meals with wholesome ingredients and better-for-you baking recipes. Her most recent book is *Supergrains*. She has worked for numerous magazines, including *Delicious*, *Australian Good Taste*, *Belle*, *Fresh*, *Recipes+*, *Healthy Food Guide*, *Super Food Ideas*, and *Weight Watchers*, and on cookbooks including *Everyday* and *Holiday* by Bill Granger, the Indulgence series, *The Biggest Loser Family Cookbook*, many Weight Watchers titles, and *The Low GI Vegetarian Cookbook*.

Chrissy and Philippa devised the challenge; Chrissy did all the recipe development and cooking and called in an expert tasting panel of friends (who all appreciate home baking) to compare the results; and Alan analyzed the recipes' nutrition. The control recipes were basic ones—a vanilla butter cookie and a blueberry bran muffin, both made with all-purpose (plain) flour—as we wanted the flavor of the sugar or sweetener to show through—and ▶**superfine** (▶**caster**) **sugar**. Recipes were tested in a conventional (not convection) oven.

MEASURING UP

- All teaspoons, tablespoons, and cup measures are level.
- 1 tablespoon equals 3 teaspoons (15 milliliters). Australian readers will need to replace their 20-milliliter tablespoon with 3 level teaspoons.
- Large eggs weigh 59 grams (2 ounces).

THE NUMBERS

Most nutrient-analysis software includes the amount of total ▶**car-bohydrates**, sugars, and ▶**starches** in a food or recipe, but not ▶**maltodextrins**. Therefore, the amount of maltodextrins in each of the recipes below has been calculated by subtracting the amount of sugars and starches from the total amount of carbohydrates.

If you are plugging the sugars, starches, and maltodextrins into your calculator, the figure won't exactly equal the available carbohydrates. This is because the information on the starch and maltodextrins content is not available for all ingredients used in the recipes.

VANILLA BUTTER COOKIE

This classic vanilla butter cookie is perfect for a challenge like this, because the ingredients include 2 tablespoons (30 ml) of milk. This meant that when we substituted liquid sweeteners for the superfine (caster) sugar, we could leave out the milk to allow for the added liquid; thus, the consistency of the batter remained similar for all the cookies we tested.

PREPARATION TIME: 25 minutes (including chilling time)
BAKING TIME: 18 to 20 minutes
MAKES 20 COOKIES

4½ ounces (125 grams) unsalted butter (9 tablespoons), diced, at room temperature

2¾ ounces (80 grams) superfine (caster) sugar (about ½ cup)

½ teaspoon pure vanilla extract

8 ounces (225 grams) all-purpose (plain) flour (about 1⅔ cups)

½ teaspoon baking powder

2 tablespoons milk (30 ml)

1. Preheat the oven to 320°F/160°C. Line a large baking sheet with parchment (baking) paper or a Silpat baking mat.

2. In a large bowl, beat the butter, sugar, and vanilla with an electric mixer until creamy and smooth.

3. Sift the flour and baking powder together into a medium bowl. Add half the flour mixture to the creamed butter mixture and stir to combine. Add the milk and the remaining flour and stir with a wooden spoon until the mixture starts to come together. Then use clean hands to mix until a soft dough forms.

4. Roll slightly rounded tablespoons of the dough into walnut-size balls and place 1½ inches (3 centimeters) apart on the prepared baking sheet. Flatten them slightly with a fork dipped in flour. Place the baking sheet in the fridge to chill for 15 minutes.

5. Bake the cookies for 18 to 20 minutes, until light golden. Remove the cookies from the oven and transfer to a wire rack to cool completely.

6. Store in an airtight container for up to 3 to 4 days.

The result:

This recipe made a delicious, crisp, sweet cookie with a vanilla, buttery taste.

- **Appearance:** Pale, light golden, slightly textured surface with small cracks.
- **Taste:** Definitely quite sweet (7–8 out of 10), but you can really taste the vanilla coming through, as well as a lovely buttery finish. The flavor is well balanced: you can taste the sweetness, but there are no distinctive overriding tones (such as caramel, toffee, etc.).
- **Texture:** Crisp, light texture (almost shortbread-like), with a buttery crumb. This was the crispest out of all the cookies.
- **The numbers (per cookie):** 103 calories/430 kilojoules; 1.3 g protein; 5.4 g fat (includes 3.5 g saturated fat); 12.3 g available carbohydrate (includes 8.2 g starch and 4.1 g sugars); 0.4 g fiber
- **Estimated glycemic index (recipe):** 68
- **Estimated glycemic load (per cookie):** 8.3

USING RICE SYRUP (RICE MALT SYRUP)

Replace the superfine (caster) sugar with ⅓ cup (3½ ounces/ 100 grams) ▶**rice syrup**. Omit the milk in step 3.

The result:

Substituting rice syrup for sugar produced a good-looking cookie but with a disappointing, bland taste with no obvious "sugar" flavors coming through.

- **Appearance:** This was possibly the best-looking of all the cookies, with a beautiful, even, light golden color and a smooth surface.
- **Taste:** Sadly, looks did not equal taste. It had a rather nondescript flavor with no obvious sweet tones, and it tasted quite floury. The taste team made comments such as: "It needs more sugar."
- **Texture:** It had a crisp outer texture, with a softer, slightly crumbly, inner texture.
- **The numbers (per cookie):** 103 calories/430 kilojoules; 1.3 g protein; 5.4 g fat (includes 3.4 g saturated fat); 12.1 g available carbohydrate (includes 8.2 g starch; 2.3 g maltodextrins; 1.6 g sugars); 0.4 g fiber

- ***Estimated glycemic index (recipe):*** 79
- ***Estimated glycemic load (per cookie):*** 9.5

USING AGAVE NECTAR (AGAVE SYRUP)

Replace the superfine (caster) sugar with ⅓ cup (3¼ ounces/ 95 grams) ▶**agave nectar/syrup**. Omit the milk in step 3.

The result:
Overall, this cookie had a lovely golden color and caramelized flavor, but the texture was dense and heavy.

- ***Appearance:*** The cookies had a relatively deep golden color with a very smooth surface.
- ***Taste:*** A quite sweet-tasting cookie; we did not really taste the vanilla or butter, but it did have a lovely, deep caramel, almost toffeelike, flavor.
- ***Texture:*** It was quite a dense cookie, a little on the heavy side. It did not have a light crumb, and it was not crisp.
- ***The numbers (per cookie):*** 101 calories/424 kilojoules; 1.3 g protein; 5.4 g fat (includes 3.4 g saturated fat); 11.9 g available carbohydrate (includes 8.2 g starch; 0.4 g maltodextrins; 3.3 g sugars); 0.4 g fiber
- ***Estimated glycemic index (recipe):*** 55
- ***Estimated glycemic load (per cookie):*** 6.5

USING HONEY

Replace the superfine (caster) sugar with ⅓ cup (4 ounces/ 115 grams) ▶**honey**. Omit the milk in step 3.

The result:
Overall, this was a deliciously golden cookie with a slightly dense texture and a fragrant, sweet aroma.

- ***Appearance:*** This cookie had an even golden color and a smooth surface.
- ***Taste:*** The taste is fragrant, almost slightly floral, and quite sweet (7–8 out of 10). However, you could not taste the vanilla at all.
- ***Texture:*** Like all the other cookies made with a liquid sweetener, it had a slightly doughy and dense texture, with a very soft crumb.

- **The numbers (per cookie):** 105 calories/438 kilojoules; 1.3 g protein; 5.4 g fat (includes 3.4 g saturated fat); 13 g available carbohydrate (includes 8.2 g starch; 4.8 g sugars); 0.4 g fiber
- **Estimated glycemic index (recipe):** 68
- **Estimated glycemic load (per cookie):** 8.8

USING A STEVIA-ERYTHRITOL BLEND (Stevia for Baking brand)

Replace the superfine (caster) sugar with ¼ cup (1¼ ounces/ 35 grams) Stevia for Baking.

The result:

Overall, this was the taste team's least favorite cookie. They reported that it did not look very attractive, and it had a lingering, slightly metallic aftertaste.

- **Appearance:** This cookie had a quite pale, textured, and slightly uneven surface, did not rise evenly, and did not brown very much. It just wasn't as golden or beautiful as the others.
- **Taste:** On first bite, the taste was quite pleasant and not overly sweet, but then came the follow-up—a lingering, very sweet, slightly bitter aftertaste on the tongue and the front palate. You could not really identify the vanilla or butter flavors—the whole point of making a vanilla butter cookie.
- **Texture:** It had a soft, crumbly, almost cakelike texture.
- **The numbers (per cookie):** 94 calories/394 kilojoules; 1.3 g protein; 5.4 g fat (includes 3.5 g saturated fat); 10 g available carbohydrate (includes 8.3 g starch; 1.5 g maltodextrins; 0.2 g sugars); 0.4 g fiber
- **Estimated glycemic index (recipe):** 76
- **Estimated glycemic load (per cookie):** 8.1

USING DEMERARA SUGAR

Replace the superfine (caster) sugar with ⅓ cup (2½ ounces/ 70 grams) ▶demerara sugar.

The result:

For flavor, this was definitely the team's favorite cookie. It was not the prettiest to look at, "but it was by far the most interesting," says Chrissy, "with a delicious caramel flavor, the slight crunch of sugar crystals, and a lovely crisp texture."

- ***Appearance:*** It had a slightly cracked, uneven surface and was a little browner than the others due to the color of the sugar. The sugar crystals were visible in the cookie.
- ***Taste:*** With a delicious, slightly caramel flavor, this was a sweet cookie but not overpoweringly so, and the flavors seemed balanced. You could taste the sugar, but you could also really taste the cookie's vanilla and buttery tones.
- ***Texture:*** It had a crisp texture with a lovely crumb. The sugar crystals gave it a slight crunch.
- ***The numbers (per cookie):*** 97 calories/407 kilojoules; 1.3 g protein; 5.4 g fat (includes 3.5 g saturated fat); 10.8 g available carbohydrate (includes 8.2 g starch; 2.6 g sugars); 0.4 g fiber
- ***Estimated glycemic index (recipe):*** 67
- ***Estimated glycemic load (per cookie):*** 7.2

USING COCONUT SUGAR

Replace the superfine (caster) sugar with ⅓ cup (1¾ ounces/ 50 grams) ▶coconut sugar.

The result:

This was a mild-tasting cookie with a very subtle toffee flavor. It did have a lovely, crisp texture and golden color.

- ***Appearance:*** Due to the rich brown color of the coconut sugar, this cookie had a lovely golden-brown color, and little specks of coconut sugar were still visible in the cookie, as coconut sugar is quite coarse and crumbly. The cookie had a slightly cracked surface.
- ***Taste:*** It had a subtle caramel-toffee flavor, but not as sweet (about a 5 out of 10) as those made with with demerara or superfine (caster) sugar. A slight hint of the vanilla came through, but overall, it was not a strong-tasting cookie.
- ***Texture:*** This was quite a crisp cookie: the sugar crystals give a very slight crunch, but only a little.
- ***The numbers (per cookie):*** 97 calories/406 kilojoules; 1.3 g protein; 5.4 g fat (includes 3.4 g saturated fat); 10.8 g available carbohydrate (includes 8.2 g starch; 0.6 g maltodextrins; 2.0 g sugars); 0.4 g fiber
- ***Estimated glycemic index (recipe):*** 65
- ***Estimated glycemic load (per cookie):*** 7

USING XYLITOL

Replace the superfine (caster) sugar with 3 tablespoons ▶**xylitol**.

The result:

This was a blond, nondescript cookie with a slightly sweet taste and a crumbly soft texture.

- **Appearance:** Quite pale. This cookie did not brown much during cooking, even when given a little extra time in the oven. It had a slightly uneven, cracked surface.
- **Taste:** This was a very neutral-tasting cookie. It was not particularly sweet, and there were no distinctive flavors coming through. It was not unpleasant and did not have any bitter aftertaste, but it was indistinctive—not what you would expect when you have gone to the bother of baking cookies.
- **Texture:** This was slightly soft and crumbly, almost cakelike, and somewhat similar to the cookie baked with stevia.
- **The numbers (per cookie):** 95 calories/398 kilojoules; 1.3 g protein; 5.4 g fat (includes 3.4 g saturated fat); 10.2 g available carbohydrate; 8.2 g starch and 2.0 g sugars); 0.8 g fiber
- **Estimated glycemic index (recipe):** 58
- **Estimated glycemic load (per cookie):** 5.9

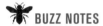 **BUZZ NOTES**

Chrissy's Tips for Cookie Makers

"For successful home-baked cookies, it is generally best to use the sweetener listed in the ingredients rather than substitute. Sometimes substituting works; very often it doesn't, or it doesn't give you the outcome you were expecting, because the cooking chemistry has changed. If you enjoy experimenting, then have fun. If you need to fill the cookie jar or want to impress, follow the recipe."

BLUEBERRY BRAN MUFFIN

*We chose a classic blueberry muffin recipe to look at the effect of different sugars and sweeteners on flavor, texture, and rise. Because we like to encourage people to try "better-for-you" baking recipes, we added some oat bran to boost the ▶**fiber** content and lower the overall GI value. Before you start baking, here are a couple of tips from Chrissy to get the best possible result. First of all, stir the blueberries into the dry ingredients, rather than adding them at the end, to prevent them from sinking to the bottom once baked. Second, don't overmix: to prevent muffins from becoming tough, stir the mixture until it is only just combined.*

PREPARATION TIME: 15 minutes
BAKING TIME: 18 to 20 minutes
MAKES 12 MUFFINS

10½ ounces (300 grams) all-purpose (plain) flour (2¼ cups)

4 teaspoons baking powder

½ teaspoon ground cinnamon

¾ cup (5¾ ounces/165 grams) superfine (caster) sugar (¾ cup)

⅓ cup (1¼ ounces/35 grams) oat bran

7 ounces (200 grams) fresh or frozen blueberries (1¼ cups)

2 large eggs

⅓ cup (2½ fluid ounces/80 ml) sunflower or other neutral vegetable oil

¾ cup (6 fluid ounces/185 ml) milk

1. Preheat the oven to 380°F/190°C. Line a 12-hole, ½-cup capacity muffin tray with paper liners.

2. Sift the flour, baking powder, and cinnamon into a large bowl. Add the sugar and oat bran and stir to combine. Stir in the blueberries.

3. Whisk the eggs, oil, and milk together in a large pitcher. Add the wet ingredients to the dry ingredients and stir until just combined (do not overmix).

4. Divide the mixture between the prepared muffin holes. Bake for 18 to 20 minutes, until golden. Transfer the muffins to a wire rack to cool.

5. These muffins are best eaten on the day they are made, but they do freeze well. Wrap individually in plastic wrap to freeze.

The result:

This recipe made a very consistent, light-textured, sweet muffin that was an all-round crowd pleaser, but it did not have much "personality," to use Chrissy's term.

- **Appearance:** This muffin had a very smooth, light golden-brown surface with only a few small cracks. It required the full 20 minutes baking time to become golden.
- **Taste:** It was quite a sweet muffin ("8 out of 10 if you're rating it") with a hint of the cinnamon. The sweetness was a nice contrast to the tart blueberries, and the muffin tasted quite balanced with its range of flavors. However, the sugar taste was rather one-dimensional and lacked character.
- **Texture:** It had a soft crumb with a light and almost fluffy texture. It was in no way heavy or dense, even with the addition of bran.
- **The numbers (per muffin):** 240 calories/1,005 kilojoules; 5.1 g protein; 8.3 g fat (includes 1.4 g saturated fat); 36 g available carbohydrate (19.7 g starch; 16.3 g sugars); 1.8 g fiber
- **Estimated glycemic index (recipe):** 65
- **Estimated glycemic load (per muffin):** 23

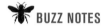 **BUZZ NOTES**

Substituting tip

When using a liquid sweetener (such as ▶**honey**), reduce the overall liquid content of recipe by approximately 1 tablespoon per ⅓ cup of liquid sweetener.

USING RICE SYRUP (RICE MALT SYRUP)

Replace the superfine (caster) sugar with ¾ cup (8 ounces/225 g) ▶**rice syrup**. Add the rice syrup to the wet ingredients in step 3; reduce the amount of milk to 4¾ fluid ounces/145 milliliters (about ½ cup plus 1½ tablespoons).

The result:

Overall, this was a deep golden crisp muffin, with a disappointing bland taste and rather heavy texture. Like the rice syrup cookie, it tasted as if it "needed more sweetness."

- **Appearance:** This muffin had an even golden surface, and it browned quickly in the oven, requiring only 18 minutes baking time. On cooling, the surface became crisp.

- **Taste:** As with the rice syrup cookie, looks were deceiving. This muffin's perfect surface was not a reflection of its taste. The flavor was very mild, almost bland, and you could not really taste any of the key blueberry or oat flavors. Even the cinnamon seemed to be lost.
- **Texture:** It had a crisp, hard surface with a dense, almost rubbery inner texture and did not have a soft crumb.
- **The numbers (per muffin):** 245 calories/1,026 kilojoules; 5.3 g protein; 8.1 g fat (includes 1.4 g saturated fat); 37 g available carbohydrate (19.7 g starch; 9.2 g maltodextrins; 8.1 g sugars); 1.8 g fiber
- **Estimated glycemic index (recipe):** 78
- **Estimated glycemic load (per muffin):** 29

USING AGAVE NECTAR (AGAVE SYRUP)

Replace the superfine (caster) sugar with ¾ cup (7½ ounces/210 grams) ▶agave nectar/syrup. Add the agave nectar to the wet ingredients in step 3, and reduce the amount of milk to 4¾ fluid ounces /145 milliliters (about ½ cup plus 1½ tablespoons).

The result:

Overall, this was a deep-golden-colored muffin with a caramel taste and slightly dense texture. Its aroma was sweeter than its taste.

- **Appearance:** This muffin was a deep golden brown with a smooth surface; however, the top of the muffins tended to peak a little, rather than rising evenly. It only required 18 minutes baking time.
- **Taste:** It was sweet and aromatic to smell, with a deep caramel, "golden syrupy" taste, but you could not taste the cinnamon.
- **Texture:** Compared to the superfine (caster) sugar control, it was not as light and had a slightly dense texture. It was not rubbery, however, nor as dense as the muffin made with rice syrup.
- **The numbers (per muffin):** 240 calories/1,002 kilojoules; 5.0 g protein; 8.2 g fat (includes 1.4 g saturated fat); 36 g available carbohydrate (19.7 g starch; 1.9 g maltodextrins; 14.4 g sugars); 1.8 g fiber
- **Estimated glycemic index (recipe):** 49
- **Estimated glycemic load (per muffin):** 17

USING HONEY

Replace the superfine (caster) sugar with ¾ cup (9¼ ounces/260 grams) ▶**honey**. Add the honey to the wet ingredients in step 3, and reduce the amount of milk to 4¾ fluid ounces/145 milliliters (about ½ cup plus 1½ tablespoons).

The result:
Overall, this was an aromatic muffin that rose well and had a slightly aerated texture.

- *Appearance:* This was a golden muffin with a slightly uneven color. As with agave syrup, the muffins rose quite high and had a tendency to dome or peak slightly in the middle rather than rising evenly.
- *Taste:* The aroma was very fragrant, especially straight out of the oven, but, like the muffins made with agave, it did not taste as sweet as it smelled, nor was it as sweet as the superfine (caster) sugar muffin.
- *Texture:* As with the other muffins made with liquid sweeteners, these were not as light in texture as the superfine (caster) sugar control muffin. There were also air holes throughout. They did have a soft crumb, especially compared with the muffins made using rice syrup.
- *The numbers (per muffin):* 254 calories/1,061 kilojoules; 5.0 g protein; 8.1 g fat (includes 1.4 g saturated fat); 40 g available carbohydrate (19.7 g starch; 20.3 g sugars); 1.8 g fiber
- *Estimated glycemic index (recipe):* 65
- *Estimated glycemic load (per muffin):* 26

USING SOFT BROWN SUGAR

Replace the superfine (caster) sugar with ¾ cup (5¾ ounces/165 grams) firmly packed soft ▶**brown sugar**.

The result:
Overall, this was a good sugar substitute for the superfine (caster) sugar if you like the strong caramel tones of brown sugar. The flavor balanced well with the blueberries.

- *Appearance:* This was a good-looking, deep-golden-brown muffin with a smooth surface and a few small cracks. It rose and browned evenly.

- **Taste:** It had delicious caramel tones, almost toffeelike, but tended to lose the flavor of the cinnamon, as the sugar's flavor was quite dominant. This was quite a sweet muffin, very much like the superfine (caster) sugar control. If you had to put a number on it, probably an 8 out of 10.
- **Texture:** This muffin had a lovely, soft, light crumb, similar in texture to the superfine (caster) sugar control.
- **The numbers (per muffin):** 240 calories/1,005 kilojoules; 5.1 g protein; 8.3 g fat (includes 1.4 g saturated fat); 36 g available carbohydrate (19.7 g starch; 16.3 g sugars); 1.8 g fiber
- **Estimated glycemic index (recipe):** 65
- **Estimated glycemic load (per muffin):** 23

USING DEMERARA SUGAR

Replace the superfine (caster) sugar with ¾ cup (5½ ounces/155 g) ▶**demerara sugar**.

The result:

This muffin was definitely a favorite. Once again, looks can be deceiving. Here, the uneven surface was no reflection of its taste. It was probably the muffin with the most interesting flavor and texture.

- **Appearance:** This muffin had a slightly bumpy, uneven surface but did turn an even golden brown. The coarse sugar crystals were still visible on the surface.
- **Taste:** As with the cookies, the demerara muffins won hands down on taste. It had a soft caramel flavor and was quite sweet, but you could still taste a hint of cinnamon, a lovely contrast to the tart blueberries. Its taste was not one-dimensional but interesting and complex compared with those made with other sugars and sweeteners (including the control).
- **Texture:** It had a soft, light crumb but also the contrast of the slight crunch of the sugar crystals, even after baking.
- **The numbers (per muffin):** 237 calories/991 kilojoules; 5.1 g protein; 8.3 g fat (includes 1.4 g saturated fat); 35 g available carbohydrate (19.6 g starch; 15.4 g sugars); 1.8 g fiber
- **Estimated glycemic index (recipe):** 62
- **Estimated glycemic load (per muffin):** 22

USING COCONUT SUGAR

Replace the superfine (caster) sugar with ¾ cup (4½ ounces/125 g) firmly packed ▶**coconut sugar**.

The result:

Overall, substituting coconut sugar could be perfect for people who prefer a slightly less sweet-tasting muffin.

- *Appearance:* Coconut sugar tends to form small lumps, which are hard to break down completely on stirring. So, once baked, the muffin wound up with small pockets of molten sugar on the surface. It had a deep golden color, similar to the muffin made with soft brown sugar.

- *Taste:* In terms of flavor, coconut sugar is quite a mild-tasting sugar with a subtle caramel taste. As this sugar is not nearly as sweet as regular brown sugar, we could still taste the cinnamon—the sugar did not overpower it.

- *Texture:* The muffin had a nice texture, soft crumb, and visible pockets of melted sugar.

- *The numbers (per muffin):* 227 calories/948 kilojoules; 5.1 g protein; 8.3 g fat (includes 1.4 g saturated fat); 33 g available carbohydrate (19.7 g starch; 2.8 g maltodextrins; 10.5 g sugars); 1.8 g fiber

- *Estimated glycemic index (recipe):* 65

- *Estimated glycemic load (per muffin):* 20

USING A MONK FRUIT WITH ERYTHRITOL SWEETENER
(Norbu brand)

Replace the superfine (caster) sugar with ½ cup (3¾ ounces/110 g) Norbu.

The result:

Although this muffin was no comparison to those made with the superfine (caster) sugar control for taste or texture, it may do the trick for anyone looking for a low-calorie muffin. By substituting Norbu for regular sugar, you can save 50 calories (210 kilojoules).

- *Appearance:* Lumpy, bumpy, and quite granular in appearance, it was the least golden of all the muffins and browned unevenly. It did not rise nearly as much as the other muffins.

- **Taste:** Initially it had quite a bland, mild taste, but this was followed by a slightly artificial sweetness on top of the palate, as all alternative, ▸**nonnutritive sweeteners** tend to have. This intense sweetness then lingered.
- **Texture:** It had quite a dense, heavy texture with a tough crumb. The top of the muffin got quite hard on cooling.
- **The numbers (per muffin):** 190 calories/795 kilojoules; 5.1 g protein; 8.3 g fat (includes 1.4 g saturated fat); 23 g available carbohydrate (19.7 g starch; 0.6 g maltodextrins; 2.7 g sugars); 1.8 g fiber
- **Estimated glycemic index (recipe):** 64
- **Estimated glycemic load (per muffin):** 17

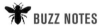 **BUZZ NOTES**

Chrissy's Tips for Muffin Makers

"I found the darker sugars such as soft brown, demerara, and coconut provided more complexity of flavor. Soft brown sugar tended to overpower the other flavors in the muffins, but it had a lovely texture, like superfine (caster) sugar, on baking. The more granulated sugars (demerara and coconut) were not visually as perfect but provided a nice textural contrast. Demerara seems to have the best flavor profile, whereas coconut is a milder, not overly sweet sugar.

"The liquid sweeteners all tended to result in muffins that rose more and domed or peaked slightly in the middle. Texture-wise, they were a little more dense and did not have as soft a crumb. Other than rice syrup, they produced a fragrant aroma and taste. Rice syrup was my least favorite, because it produced a muffin that was bland and boring with a very heavy, rubbery texture."

NOTES

1 Alyssa Crittenden, PhD, "How Honey Helped to Make Us Human," *GI News*, January 2013: http://ginews.blogspot.com/2013_01_01_archive.html.

2 C. Fitch and K. S. Keim, "Position of the Academy of Nutrition and Dietetics: Use of Nutritive and Nonnutritive Sweeteners," *Journal of the Academy of Nutrition and Dietetics* 112, no. 5 (2012): 739, doi:10.1016/j.jand.2012.03.00.

3 "WHO Opens Public Consultation on Draft Sugars Guideline: Note for Media," World Health Organization, March 5, 2014, http://www.who.int/mediacentre/news/notes/2014/consultation-sugar-guideline.

4 Brian Wansink, Aner Tal, and Adam Brumberg, "Ingredient-based Food Fears and Avoidance: Antecedents and Antidotes," *Food Quality and Preference* 38 (December 2014): 40–48, http://www.sciencedirect.com/science/article/pii/S0950329314001128.

5 "Generally Recognized as Safe (GRAS)" U.S. Food and Drug Administration, last modified July 14, 2014, http://www.fda.gov/food/IngredientspackagingLabeling/GRAS.

6 Fiona S. Atkinson, RD, Kaye Foster-Powell, RD, and Jennie C. Brand-Miller, PhD, "International Tables of Glycemic Index and Glycemic Load Values: 2008," *Diabetes Care* 31, no. 12 (December 2008): 2281–83.
   "Search for the Glycemic Index," The University of Sydney, last modified August 8, 2014, http://www.glycemicindex.com/foodSearch.php.

7 Mary Beth O'Leary, "The Dark Side of Artificial Sweeteners," *EurekAlert!* press release, July 10, 2013, http://www.eurekalert.org/pub_releases/2013-07/cp-tds070313.php.

8 Richard D. Mattes and Barry M. Popkin, "Nonnutritive Sweetener Consumption in Humans: Effects on Appetite and Food Intake and Their Putative Mechanisms," *The American Journal of Clinical Nutrition* 89, no. 1 (January 2009), 1–14.

9 Kommi Kalpana, Priti Rishi Lal, Doddipalli Lakshmi Kusuma, and Gulshan Lal Khanna, "The Effects of Ingestion of Sugarcane Juice and Commercial Sports Drinks on Cycling Performance of Athletes in Comparison to Plain Water," *Asian Journal of Sports Medicine* 4, no. 3 (September 2013): 181–89.

10 "Introduction," *Acta Physiologica Scandinavica* 44 (1958): 7–27, doi:10.1111/j.1748-1716.1958.tb01658.x.

11 Hend Hassan and Ali Ganbi, "Production of Nutritious High Quality Date (*Phoenix dactylifera*) Fruits Syrup (Dibs) by Using Some Novel Technological Approaches," *Journal of Applied Sciences Research* 8, no. 3 (2012): 1524–38. http://www.aensiweb.com/old/jasr/jasr/2012/1524-1538.pdf.

12 "DRAFT Guidance for Industry: Ingredients Declared as Evaporated Cane Juice; Draft Guidance," U.S. Food and Drug Administration, October 2009, last modified July 9, 2014, http://www.fda.gov/food/guidanceregulation/guidancedocumentsregulatoryinformation/labelingnutrition/ucm181491.htm.

13 Sue Shepherd and Peter Gibson, *The Complete Low-FODMAP Diet: A Revolutionary Plan for Managing IBS and Other Digestive Disorders* (New York: The Experiment, 2013).

14 John L. Sievenpiper, Russell J. de Souza, Arash Mirrahimi, Matthew E. Yu, Amanda J. Carleton, Joseph Beyene, Laura Chiavaroli, Marco Di Buono, Alexandra L. Jenkins, Lawrence A. Leiter, Thomas M. S. Wolever, Cyril W. C. Kendall, and David J. A. Jenkins, "Effect of Fructose on Body Weight in Controlled Feeding Trials: A Systematic Review and Meta-analysis," *Annals of Internal Medicine* 156, no. 4 (February 21, 2012): 291–304.

15 David Katz, "Food for Thought: Sugar, Diabetes and Why the State of Our Health Is Not About Any One Thing," *GI News*, October 1, 2013: http://ginews.blogspot.com/2013/10/food-for-thought.html.

16 GI Group, "Q&A with Jennie Brand-Miller," *GI News*, May 1, 2014: http://ginews.blogspot.com/2014/05/q-with-jennie-brand-miller.html.

17 Peter Hull, *Glucose Syrups: Technology and Applications* (West Sussex, UK: John Wiley & Sons, 2010): 1.

18 William Moore, "On the Production of Sugar from the Starch of Wheat, and of Potatoes, by the Agency of Sulphuric Acid," *The Philosophical Magazine* 40, no. 172 (August 1812): 14.

19 Jennie Brand-Miller, *The Low-GI Eating Plan for an Optimal Pregnancy: The Authoritative Science-Based Nutrition Guide for Mother and Baby* (New York: The Experiment, 2013): 73–74.

20 "Anzac Biscuit Recipes," Australian War Memorial Encyclopedia, accessed August 27, 2014, http://www.awm.gov.au/encyclopedia/anzac/biscuit/recipe.

21 J. H. Galloway, *The Sugar Cane Industry: An Historical Geography from Its Origins to 1914* (New York: Cambridge University Press, 1989): 20.

22 Richard Kahn and John L. Sievenpiper, "Dietary Sugar and Body Weight: Have We Reached a Crisis in the Epidemic of Obesity and Diabetes? We Have, but the Pox on Sugar Is Overwrought and Overworked," *Diabetes Care* 37, no. 4 (April 2014), doi:10.2337/dc13-2506.

23 Food and Agriculture Organization of the United Nations, "Appendix II. Draft Revised Standard for Honey," *Joint FAO/WHO Food Standard Programme Codex Alimentarius Commission*, Twenty-Fourth Session, Geneva, July 2–7, 2001. http://www.fao.org/docrep/meeting/005/x4616e/x4616e0b.htm.

24 Jerónimo Lobo, *A Voyage to Abyssinia*, translated by Samuel Johnson (London: Elliot and Kay, and C Elliott, Edinburgh, 1789).

25 Stefanie Brunner, Ines Holub, Stephan Theis, Andrea Gostner, Ralph Melcher, Petra Wolf, Ulrike Amann-Gassner, Wolfgang Scheppach, and Hans Hauner, "Metabolic Effects of Replacing Sucrose by Isomaltulose in Subjects with Type 2 Diabetes: A Randomized Double-blind Trial," *Diabetes Care* 35, no. 6 (June 2012): 1249–51, doi:10.2337/dc11-1485.

26 Charles Perry, "Manna," in *The Oxford Companion to Food*, 2nd ed. (Oxford, UK: 2006).

27 Bernd Heinrich, "Maple Sugaring by Red Squirrels," *Journal of Mammalogy* 73, no. 1 (1992): 51–54.

28 James Smith, *Remarkable Occurrences in the Life and Travels of Col. James Smith, (Now a Citizen of Bourbon County, Kentucky) During His Captivity with the Indians, in the Years 1755, '56, '57, '58, & '59* (Lexington, KY: John Bradford, on Main Street, 1799).

29 GI Group, "Q&A with Jennie Brand-Miller," *GI News*, February 1, 2014: http://ginews.blogspot.com/2014/02/q-with-jennie-brand-miller.html.

30 Peter Felker, "Mesquite Flour: New Life for an Ancient Staple," *Gastronomica: The Journal of Critical Food Studies* 5, no. 2 (Spring 2005): 85–89.

31 M. K. Wilken and B. A. Satiroff, "Pilot Study of 'Miracle Fruit' to Improve Food Palatability for Patients Receiving Chemotherapy," *Clinical Journal of Oncology Nursing* 16, no. 5 (October 2012): E173–77, http://www.ncbi.nlm.nih.gov/pubmed/23022943.

32 Daniel Engber, "The Quest for a Natural Sugar Substitute," *The New York Times*, January 1, 2014, http://www.nytimes.com/2014/01/05/magazine/the-quest-for-a-natural-sugar-substitute.html.

33 Walter T. Swingle, "*Momordica grosvenori* sp. nov.: The Source of the Chinese Lo Han Kuo," *Journal of the Arnold Arboretum* 22 (1941): 197–203.

34 Mrinal Roy, "Innovation: The Case of Cane Special Sugars" (article presented at the Symposium on Agriculture, October 29–31, 2003), http://www.mchagric.org/php/int_main.php?rub=130.

35 Christopher Gardner, Judith Wylie-Rosett, Samuel S. Gidding, Lyn M. Steffen, Rachel K. Johnson, Diane Reader, Alice H. Lichtenstein, American Heart Association Nutrition Committee of the Council on Nutrition, Physical Activity and Metabolism, Council on Arteriosclerosis, Thrombosis and Vascular Biology, Council on Cardiovascular Disease in the Young, and the American Diabetes Association, "Nonnutritive Sweeteners: Current Use and Health Perspectives: A Scientific Statement from the American Heart Association and the American Diabetes Association," *Circulation* 126 (2012): 509–19, doi:10.1161/CIR.0b013e31825c42ee.

36 "National Organic Program," United States Department of Agriculture Agricultural Marketing Service website, last modified October 17, 2012, http://tinyurl.com/5vanen.

37 "Sugar Consumption at a Crossroad," (Zurich, Switzerland: Credit Suisse AG, September 2013).

38 Katherine Beals and David Ropa, "Effects of Processing on the Pollen and Nutrient Content of Honey," National Honey Board, accessed August 28, 2014, http://www.honey.com/images/uploads/general/Beals_abstract_on_Effects_of_Processing.pdf.

39 "Artificial Sweeteners and Cancer," National Cancer Institute at the National Institutes of Health website, last modified August 5, 2009, http://www.cancer.gov/cancertopics/factsheet/Risk/artificial-sweeteners.

40 "The Inventor of Saccharine," *Scientific American* 55, no. 3 (July 17, 1886): 36.

41 Noah Strycker, *The Thing with Feathers: The Surprising Lives of Birds and What They Reveal About Being Human* (New York: Riverhead Books, 2014): 92.

42 Joint FAO/WHO Expert Committee on Food Additives, *Compendium of Food Additive Specifications* (Rome, Italy: FAO, 2007): 61.

43 Ian Hemphill, *The Spice and Herb Bible*, 2nd ed. (Toronto, Ontario: Robert Rose, 2006): 479–81.

44 Harold McGee, *On Food and Cooking: The Science and Lore of the Kitchen* (New York: Scribner, 2004).

45 Hannah Glasse, *The Art of Cookery, Made Plain and Easy* (London: 1774).

46 Mani Niall, *Sweet!: From Agave to Turbinado, Home Baking with Every Kind of Natural Sugar and Sweetener with More Than 100 Recipes* (Philadelphia, PA: Da Capo Press, 2008): 13.

47 "Vegetables Nutrition Facts," U.S. Food and Drug Administration, January 1, 2008, http://www.fda.gov/downloads/Food/GuidanceRegulation/ucm063477.pdf. "Vegetable Nutrition Facts," Wegmans.com, September 7, 2004, accessed August 28, 2014, http://www.wegmans.com/pdf/nutrition/vegetables.pdf. NUTTAB 2010 Online Searchable Database, accessed August 28, 2014, http://www.foodstandards.gov.au/science/monitoringnutrients/nutrientables/nuttab/Pages/default.aspx.

48 E. G. Engleman, J. Lankton, and B. Lankton, "Granulated Sugar as Treatment for Hiccups in Conscious Patients," *New England Journal of Medicine* 285, no. 26 (December 23, 1971): 1489.

49 Quanhe Yang, Zefeng Zhang, Edward W. Gregg, W. Dana Flanders, Robert Merritt, and Frank B. Hu, "Added Sugar Intake and Cardiovascular Diseases Mortality Among US Adults," *JAMA Internal Medicine* 174, no. 4 (April 2014): 516–24, doi:10.1001/jamainternmed.2013.13563.

50 U.S. Department of Agriculture and U.S. Department of Health and Human Services, *Dietary Guidelines for Americans 2010*, 7th ed. (Washington, DC: U.S. Government Printing Office, 2010): i.

51 R. K. Johnson, L. J. Appel, M. Brands, B. V. Howard, M. Lefevre, R. H. Lustig, F. Sacks, L. M. Steffen, J. Wylie-Rosett, American Heart Association Nutrition Committee of the Council on Nutrition, Physical Activity, and Metabolism and the Council on Epidemiology and Prevention, "Dietary Sugars Intake and Cardiovascular Health: A Scientific Statement from the American Heart Association," *Circulation* 120, no. 11 (September 2009): 1011–20. doi:10.1161/CIRCULATIONAHA.109.192627.

52 Ryan O'Malley and Allison MacMunn, "Position of Academy of Nutrition and Dietetics: Safely Enjoy Sweetened Foods Within a Healthful Eating Plan," Academy of Nutrition and Dietetics press release, May 1, 2012, http://www.eatright.org/Media/content.aspx?id=6442469620#.U4A61Ch-iSo.

53 Michael Pollan, "Unhappy Meals," *The New York Times* (January 28, 2007), http://www.nytimes.com/2007/01/28/magazine/28nutritionism.t.html.

54 Ministério da Saúde, Secretaria de Atenção à Saúde, Departamento de Atenção Básica, and Coordenação Geral de Alimentação e Nutrição, *Guia Alimentar Para a População Brasileira*, 2014, http://www.foodpolitics.com/wp-content/uploads/Brazils-Dietary-Guidelines_2014.pdf.

55 Sam Z. Sun and Mark W. Empie, "Fructose Metabolism in Humans—What Isotopic Tracer Studies Tell Us," *Nutrition & Metabolism* 9, no. 89 (October 2012), doi:10.1186/1743-7075-9-89.

56 A. Deshpande and A. R. Jadad, "The Impact of Polyol-Containing Chewing Gums on Dental Caries: A Systematic Review of Original Randomized Controlled Trials and Observational Studies," *The Journal of the American Dental Association* 139, no. 12 (December 2008): 1602–14, http://www.ncbi.nlm.nih.gov/pubmed/19047666.

57 H. Hauner, A. Bechthold, H. Boeing, A. Brönstrup, A. Buyken, E. Leschik-Bonnet, J. Linseisen, M. Schulze, D. Strohm, G. Wolfram, and the German Nutrition Society, "Evidence-Based Guideline of the German Nutrition Society: Carbohydrate Intake and Prevention of Nutrition-Related Diseases," *Annals of Nutrition and Metabolism* 60, suppl. 1 (2012): 1–58, doi:10.1159/000335326.

58 V.S. Malik, B.M. Popkin, G.A. Bray, J.P. Després, W.C. Willett, F.B. Hu, "Sugar-Sweetened Beverages and Risk of Metabolic Syndrome and Type 2 Diabetes: A Meta-Analysis," *Diabetes Care* 33, no. 11 (November 2010): 2477–83, doi:10.2337/dc10-1079.

59 C. L. Gillies, K. R. Abrams, P. C. Lambert, N. J. Cooper, A. J. Sutton, R. T. Hsu, and K. Khunti, "Pharmacological and Lifestyle Interventions to Prevent or Delay Type 2 Diabetes in People with Impaired Glucose Tolerance: Systematic Review and Meta-Analysis," *BMJ* 334, no. 7588 (February 10, 2007): 299, http://www.ncbi.nlm.nih.gov/pubmed/17237299.

60 American Diabetes Association, J. P. Bantle, J. Wylie-Rosett, A. L. Albright, C. M. Apovian, N. G. Clark, M. J. Franz, B. J. Hoogwerf, A. H. Lichtenstein, E. Mayer-Davis, A. D. Mooradian, M. L. Wheeler, "Nutrition Recommendations and Interventions for Diabetes: A Position Statement of the American Diabetes Association," *Diabetes Care* 31, suppl. 1 (January 2008): S61–78, doi:10.2337/dc08-S061.

61 Michael Pollan, *Food Rules: An Eater's Manual* (New York: Penguin Books, 2009).

62 Citation needed

63 Lisa Te Morenga, Simonette Mallard, and Jim Mann, "Dietary Sugars and Body Weight: Systematic Review and Meta-Analyses of Randomised Controlled Trials and Cohort Studies," *BMJ* 346 (January 2012): e7492, doi:10.1136/bmj.e7492.

APPENDIX

BRAND NAMES OF HIGH-INTENSITY, NONNUTRITIVE SWEETENERS

This is a table of the most commonly available consumer brands of ▶high-intensity, ▶nonnutritive sweeteners. We have also included products such as Aclame, because you will see this brand popping up in various published lists of alternative sweeteners, but you would be hard pressed to find it on shelves as it does not appear to be available anywhere (we have read that manufacture was discontinued as the cost of production is very high).

When selecting a sweetener, always check the ingredient list. Formulations change from time to time, and country to country. You will also find that the ingredient list for granule products looks different from the list for tablets, because tablets need additives ("binders" or "carriers") so that they stick together. Canderel (a UK brand), for example, lists its products' ingredients this way (as of mid-2014):

- *Canderel granules*—Maltodextrin, aspartame and acesulfame potassium, flavoring
- *Canderel tablets*—Lactose, aspartame and acesulfame potassium, leucine, binder: cross-linked sodium CMC (carboxy methyl cellulose), flavoring
- *Canderel Yellow granules*—Maltodextrin, sucralose 0.7%, acesulfame potassium 0.6%, flavorings
- *Canderel Yellow tablets*—Lactose (from milk), sucralose 7.3%, stabilizer: microcrystalline cellulose, flavors, binder: cross-linked sodium CMC (carboxy methyl cellulose)
- *Canderel Green granules*—Maltodextrin, steviol glycocides, natural flavorings
- *Canderel Green tablets*—Lactose (from milk), steviol glycocides, natural flavorings, carrier: cross-linked sodium CMC (carboxy methyl cellulose), anticaking agents: calcium salts of fatty acids and silicon dioxide

We hope we have captured all the readily available products, but please let us know if you find a new product you think we should know about. The best way to do this is using the "Contact" form on our website: sugarsandsweeteners.com.

BRAND NAME	NNS USED
Aclame™	Alitame
AminoSweet®	Aspartame
Assugrin® Classic	Cyclamate/saccharin
Assugrin® Premium	Cyclamate/saccharin/aspartame
Assugrin® Stevia Sweet	Stevia
Better Stevia™	Stevia
BlueSweet™	Monk fruit
Canderel®	Aspartame/acesulfame potassium
Canderel® Yellow	Sucralose
Canderel® Green	Stevia
CandyS®	Sucralose
Chuker	Cyclamate
Cologran® Sweetener Tablets	Saccharin/cyclamate
Cologran® Granulated	Aspartame
Cukren®	Sucralose
Cweet (approval expected 2014/15)	Brazzein
Enliten®	Stevia
Equal® Classic	Aspartame/acesulfame potassium
Equal® Next	Aspartame/saccharin
Equal® Original	Aspartame/acesulfame potassium
Equal® Saccharin	Saccharin
Equal® Spoonful/Equal® Measure	Aspartame/acesulfame potassium
Equal® Stevia	Stevia
Equal® Sucralose	Sucralose
EZ-Sweetz®	Sucralose
Fructevia™	Stevia
Fruit-Sweetness™	Monk fruit
Hermesetas Gold	Acesulfame potassium/aspartame
Hermesetas Granulated	Acesulfame potassium/aspartame
Hermesetas Stevia Granulated	Stevia/thaumatin
Hermesetas SteviaSweet/Stevia Liquid	Stevia
Hermesetas Tablets/Mini Sweeteners	Saccharin

[Table continues]

BRAND NAME	NNS SWEETENER(S) USED
Luo Han Guo Monk Fruit Extract	Monk fruit
Magou-V™	Monk fruit
Monk Fruit in the Raw®	Monk fruit
NatraTaste Blue™	Aspartame
NatraTaste Gold™	Sucralose
Natrena® Stevia	Stevia
Naturlose™	Tagatose
Natvia™	Stevia
Necta Sweet®	Saccharin
Nectresse®	Monk fruit
Nevella®	Sucralose
Nevella® Stevia	Stevia
Nevella® with Probiotics	Sucralose
Norbu®	Monk fruit
NovaSweet®	Cyclamate
NuStevia™	Stevia
NutraSweet®	Aspartame
Only Sweet™	Stevia
PureCircle® Alpha Stevia	Stevia
Purefruit™	Monk fruit
PureLo®	Monk fruit
PureVia®	Stevia
Pyure® Stevia	Stevia
Rebiana®	Stevia
Sanecta™	Aspartame
Silver Spoon® Sweetness & Light Granulated	Aspartame/acesulfame potassium
Silver Spoon® Sweetness & Light Tablet	Aspartame/acesulfame potassium
Skinnygirl™ Monk Fruit	Monk fruit
Skinnygirl™ Stevia	Stevia
Splenda®	Sucralose
Stevia in the Raw®	Stevia
Stevita®	Stevia
Steviva™ Blend	Stevia
Sucaryl®	Cyclamate/saccharin
Sucralean®	Sucralose
SucraLow®	Sucralose
SucraPlus™	Sucralose

BRAND NAME	NNS SWEETENER(S) USED
Sucron	Saccharin
Sugar Twin® (blue box)	Aspartame
Sugar Twin® Liquid Sweetener	Cyclamate
Sugar Twin® (yellow box)	Saccharin (US); cyclamate (Canada)
Sugarella®	Saccharin
Sugarine®	Saccharin
Sugarless	Aspartame/acesulfame potassium
Sugarless Organic Stevia	Stevia
Sugarless Sugar™	Stevia
Suitli	Cyclamate
Sukrana®	Sucralose
Sun Crystals®	Stevia
Sunett®	Acesulfame potassium
Sweet & Safe	Acesulfame potassium
Sweetex	Saccharin
SweetLeaf®	Stevia
Sweet'N Low®	Saccharin (US); cyclamate (Canada)
Sweet One®	Acesulfame potassium
Neway Sweet Sensation	Monk fruit
Sweet Twin®	Saccharin
Sweetzfree	Sucralose
Swerve®	Erythritol
Swiss Sweet®	Acesulfame potassium
Tagatesse®	Tagatose/sucralose
Talin®	Thaumatin
Tesco Everyday Value Tablet Sweeteners	Cyclamate/saccharin
Tesco Stevia	Stevia
Tesco Sucralose	Sucralose
Tesco Tablet Sweeteners	Aspartame
Triple Zero Sugar	Stevia
Truvia®	Stevia
Twinsweet™	Aspartame/acesulfame potassium
Weider Stevia Sweet®	Stevia

ACKNOWLEDGMENTS

In the beginning • The idea for this book popped out when we were answering a question from a colleague. Back in 2013, Chrissy Freer, author of the delicious *Supergrains*, quizzed us about rice syrup as magazine editors kept asking her to use it in developing recipes for "healthier" baking. "Is it actually a 'healthier' alternative to sugar or just another fashionable sweetener being touted as sugar-free and better for you?" she asked. So we wrote a piece about the current crop of celebrity sweeteners for *GI News*.

Enter our publisher Matthew Lore from The Experiment. He thought there could be a book in this, and encouraged us to expand our story into a comprehensive proposal for an A to Z guide to sugars and sweeteners. We would like to thank them both very much for the idea and the opportunity. (And no, rice syrup is not sugar-free. It is sugar: glucose in one form or another and it has a very high GI value.)

Creating the book • Molly Cavanaugh, associate editor at The Experiment, has held our hands and encouraged us throughout the whole process from tweaking the original proposal to editing the manuscript, and bringing the three of us together. During the editing process she gently (and regularly) reminded us that writing books is different from writing topical pieces for an online health newsletter and forced us to translate the science into everyday language. She has been actively involved in creating this book at every stage and she has our gratitude for all she has contributed.

We could not have asked for a better, more efficient production team at The Experiment and would specifically like to thank designer Pauline Neuwirth, cover designer Christopher Brian King, managing editor Dan O'Connor and digital publishing manager Karen Giangreco, who created the ebook. And it goes without saying that this is a much better book thanks to the eagle eyes of our copyeditor Leslie Kazan and proofreader Jeanne Tao. We also appreciate the efforts of

Jennifer Hergenroeder, Sarah Schneider, and Anne Rumberger in publicity and marketing for their constant efforts to promote the book to the wider world.

Inside the book • Numerous people who are experts in areas we are not very familiar with have shared insights and information, and generously given us permission to quote from their published works. In particular we would like to thank: Prof. Alyssa Crittenden (*The Importance of Honey Consumption in Human Evolution*); Casa de Mesquite's Peter Felker (*Mesquite Flour: New Life for an Ancient Staple*); Ian Hemphill (*The Spice and Herb Bible*, Third Edition, Robert Rose); Prof. David Katz (*Sweet Nothings, Bitter Truth*); Moses Murandu ("Use of Granulated Sugar Therapy in the Management of Sloughy or Necrotic Wounds: A PilotStudy"); John Palmer (*How to Brew: Everything You Need to Know to Brew Beer Right the First Time*); Nicole Senior (*Food Myths* and also for reading and commenting on the entire manuscript at an early stage); and Colibree's Sabra Van Dolsen who chatted to us about her experience launching agave syrup into the United States at Expo West in 1995.

Behind the scenes • Thanks to Jennie Brand-Miller for her support (and blessing) and for writing the foreword and to our many colleagues, friends and family members whose brains we picked and who read bits of manuscript and made suggestions along the way including Fiona Atkinson, Caroline Attwooll, Utku Ayhan, Mitchell Beare, Jonathon Cohen, Dr. Alan Kirkness, Kai Lin Ek, Kate McGhie, Anneka Manning, Dr. Kate Marsh, Suzy Montignac, Prof. Nic Peterson, Emma Sandall, and Catherine Saxelby.

We would also like to thank chefs Yotam Ottolenghi and Sami Tamimi, whom we have never met, but whose inspirational cookbook *Jeruslaem*, with its wonderful dressings and drizzles using a dash of traditional sweeteners like maple syrup or date syrup, deliciously reminded us how a little sugar can make the healthiest of foods (including cauliflower) not only go down, but have the troops lining up for seconds.

INDEX

Page numbers in *italics* refer to tables and figures. A-to-Z entries have not been indexed.

ABOUT THE AUTHORS

Alan Barclay, PhD, is a consultant dietitian who worked for Diabetes Australia (NSW) from 1998 to 2014. He is coauthor of *The New Glucose Revolution for Diabetes* and a member of the editorial boards of the Diabetes Australia's consumer magazine, *Conquest*, and health professional magazine, *Diabetes Management Journal*. Barclay is currently Chief Scientific Officer at the Glycemic Index Foundation.

Claudia Shwide-Slavin, MS, RD, CDE, has been a registered dietitian and a certified diabetes educator for over twenty years. She runs a clinical private practice in New York City, prior to which she set up and coordinated three diabetes centers in the NYC area. Her writing on diabetes and sweeteners has appeared in various peer-reviewed journals.

Philippa Sandall is editor of the University of Sydney Human Nutrition Unit's *GI News* newsletter (http://ginews.blogspot.com), which has more than 100,000 subscribers worldwide. She is also coauthor, with Jennie Brand-Miller, of several books in the *New York Times*-bestselling New Glucose Revolution series. A longtime book editor, she now runs her own editorial consulting agency, Philippa Sandall Publishing Services, in New South Wales, Australia.